The 360 Mama Guide to C-section Recovery

EMMA BRADLEY AND HANNAH WEST

The 360 Mama Guide to C-section Recovery

EMMA BRADLEY AND HANNAH WEST

sheldon PRESS

First published by Sheldon Press in 2025
An imprint of John Murray Press

1

A CIP catalogue record for this title is available from the British Library

Trade Paperback ISBN 9781399818353
ebook ISBN 9781399818360

Typeset by KnowledgeWorks Global Ltd.

Printed and bound in Canada

John Murray Press policy is to use papers that are natural, renewable and recyclable products and made from wood grown in sustainable forests. The logging and manufacturing processes are expected to conform to the environmental regulations of the country of origin.

John Murray Press
Carmelite House
50 Victoria Embankment
London EC4Y 0DZ

Sheldon Press
123 S. Broad St., Ste 2750
Philadelphia, PA, 19109

www.sheldonpress.co.uk

John Murray Press, part of Hodder & Stoughton Limited
An Hachette UK company

The authorised representative in the EEA is Hachette Ireland,
8 Castlecourt Centre, Dublin 15, D15 XTP3, Ireland (email: info@hbgi.ie)

For my two incredible children, who inspire me daily to do more than I thought I was capable of. Becoming your mum has changed me, changed my world and has given me a sense of confidence and purpose that I didn't have before you. – Emma

For Caspar and Otis, follow your dreams babies, you are my reason and purpose for following mine. And for my awesome husband who makes juggling life so much more enjoyable and easier to do it with. – Hannah

To The 360 Mama community, what we have built together is a wonderful example of women supporting women, of which we are extremely proud. Thank you for all of your support so far.

Contents

About The 360 Mama

The 360 Mama is made up of a team of postpartum experts who are passionate about improving the lives of mothers after pregnancy and birth. Emma, a pelvic health physiotherapist and Pilates instructor and Hannah, a soft-tissue and scar massage therapist, are both mothers themselves, and recognize the need for better support and education for modern mothers to thrive after birth.

Emma has been practising as a Chartered Physiotherapist for 15 years, with a BSc (Hons) in Physiotherapy and MSc in Sports & Exercise Medicine. Her further interest in rehabilitation and exercise led her to qualify as a Pilates Instructor with the Australian Physiotherapy & Pilates Institute, and later go on to specialize in pre-and postnatal Pilates training. Her passion to support women through pregnancy and beyond resulted in further postgraduate training in pelvic health and she is now a qualified Mummy MOT practitioner and a member of the Pelvic, Obstetric and Gynaecological Physiotherapy professional group.

Hannah qualified with a BTEC level 5 in sports and remedial massage in 2013. Passionate about women's health, she furthered her training in pregnancy and postnatal massage, abdominal scar massage and scar work for all types of scars with the UK-leading scar massage therapist and also qualified in Oncology Massage. She is also qualified in medical acupuncture. Hannah is a member of both the Complementary Health Professionals Association and a gold member of the Sports Massage Association.

Individually, Emma and Hannah both support and treat women in the postpartum period in their daily clinical roles. They were inspired to launch 360 Mama as they so frequently heard the phrase 'I wish somebody had told me this before' in relation to how to heal properly from pregnancy and birth. They know that the foundations for a successful postpartum recovery stem from simple actions that could be achievable for every person, if they were able to access the right information.

Across their platforms they strive to offer daily videos to educate people about how to take care of themselves properly after having a baby, making postpartum care accessible in a format that is easy to digest and offer tips that are easy to implement. Since launching their TikTok account they have amassed a large active following and audience across TikTok, Instagram, YouTube and Facebook and a large subscribed audience to their regular newsletter, which demonstrates the demand and desire for more information and support for Cesarean section (C-section) and postpartum recovery.

This is the book that every new parent should read to better inform their birth choices, plan for a successful recovery and feel confident to navigate the postpartum period after a C-section. As mothers themselves, they are fully aware of how demanding life as a new parent can be so hope that as you read this book you feel you've got a support team on your side, you can benefit from a community of other mothers sharing their stories and find answers to every question you have throughout your journey.

Introduction

In the UK, around one in every four birthing women (31 per cent) have a Cesarean section (C-section), but only 16 per cent of those are elective.[1,2] For those who have not prepared for this type of birth beforehand, there can often be a lack of understanding of what to expect during the operation or how to recover, which can contribute to feeling a loss of control or negative feelings surrounding the birth experience. This is why we'd like to encourage families to spend some time considering their preferences for a Caesarean birth, even if it's not their preferred birth choice. Birth is unpredictable, but planning for any eventuality can give you and your birthing partner or support network the best chance of a positive birth and successful recovery.

Unfortunately women's health is underserved worldwide. Most women get very little information from their healthcare providers after having a C-section or help with rehabilitation during their recovery. Many women report feeling very much lost, sore and unsure about what they should and shouldn't do whilst also feeling overwhelmed with having a new baby to care for.

The most frequent question we hear from mothers is 'why didn't someone tell me this sooner?' It is our hope to solve this problem with this book.

If you're currently pregnant, and preparing for a C-section birth, we recommend you start to read the book now. Knowledge is power, and good preparation can be the key to having a positive birth and postpartum experience, and ultimately mean a much better recovery both physically and mentally. Even if you think a C-section is the last thing you want and it's not part of your birth plan, reading this book can help you feel better prepared for any outcome; a worthwhile effort because birth is so unpredictable.

If you've already given birth, especially following an unplanned C-section, it's likely you'll have questions about your experience, or you may need support to process it. We've sought the advice of other birth professionals who offer their expertise throughout the book to help you address all aspects of your recovery. If you are considering future pregnancies, resolving any emotional as well as physical concerns is an important part of your recovery. When the time is right, you will benefit from all the preparation advice included in the book to plan ahead for your next birth.

We know that some of you will read this book cover to cover, while others will read chapters in isolation as you seek specific answers or according to what you need at the time. For this reason you will notice that we do repeat some important information occasionally across chapters, because we feel it is particularly relevant to that chapter and we don't want you to miss it. Recovering well from a C-section is best achieved if you take a holistic approach, so while you may have a particular interest in one of the topics, we'd encourage you to take the time to learn about all the others we've included in the book and include them in your plan. You may be surprised by how much your fitness progression is impacted by your nutrition, or how your tummy or scar appearance is affected by different massage techniques that are introduced deliberately in stages.

We've arranged the order of the chapters according to a chrono-logical timeline, supporting you from the beginning as you prepare for birth, all the way through the stages of recovery to the end. The instructions for scar care and massage and exercise advice will change as you move through healing phases and as you make progress, so we've chosen to order the chapters to follow this timeline rather than into topics. For example, some types of exercise are just not appro-priate until you are a little further along in the healing journey, but we don't want to delay you learning about the types of movement or exercise that can be started earlier on because it's an important part of that phase of recovery. The same goes for different massaging techniques for your scar – it needs to happen in the right order to get the best results.

We also really hope this book will better help others to understand about C-sections and be more compassionate to all parents, however their child was born. The pure definition of birth is 'the emergence of a baby from the body of its mother' so however you give birth, YOU did it mama. And whether you chose a C-section or not, it was the right decision in the circumstances; this was the right choice for you and your family.

Understanding what to expect during a C-section and the recovery period that follows is crucial for several reasons. It can help you feel prepared both mentally and physically for the experience, it helps to alleviate anxiety and uncertainty, can significantly improve how you feel about the birth after and enhance your recovery.

- **Mental preparation**: Knowing the steps involved during a C-section can significantly reduce stress and anxiety. It allows you to visualize the process, understand the reasoning behind each step, and mentally prepare for the birth of your child. This mental preparation is the key to a more positive birthing experience, as it helps to build confidence and give you a sense of control over the situation.
- **Physical preparation**: Understanding the physical aspects of what happens during the C-section procedure helps you to prepare your body. Being aware of the pre-operative instructions, such as fasting or hygiene measures, is important for your safety and the success of the surgery. Also knowing what physical sensations to expect during the procedure, such as pressure or tugging, can make the experience less daunting.
- **Informed decision-making**: Being well-informed about the procedure enables you to make educated decisions regarding your birth plan. This includes choices about pain management, the presence of a birth partner, and preferences like playing music or cutting the umbilical cord.
- **Emotional support**: Anticipating the emotional aspects of a C-section, such as the joy of meeting your baby and the possible feelings of detachment or disappointment due to a surgical birth, is important. Understanding and validating these emotions helps with coping with them more effectively.
- **Recovery expectations**: Knowledge about the recovery process post-C-section is vital and often where so many women feel lost. It involves understanding pain management, wound care, limitations in physical activities, and signs of complications. This awareness is essential for a smooth recovery and for reducing the risk of complications after the birth.
- **Planning for postpartum**: It can be tough recovering from a C-section and knowing what to expect helps you to put plans in place for after you leave the hospital. Ultimately this means understanding the limitations you might face in the initial weeks and working out a plan for how to overcome them. This will include things like arranging

your house so you can easily access what you need, having nutritious meals ready that don't require you to spend ages cooking them, making time for you to rest and possibly planning for help with baby or older children.

Advice for our readers

Your medical history and experience is individual to you. It's important to acknowledge that the advice in this book is of a generalist nature and cannot take into account the particular physical or medical condition of individual readers.

The information provided in this book is meant to be practical and informative, but is not intended to be a substitute for professional advice.

The information provided is not meant to replace any relationship that exists between the reader and their doctor, medical team, hospital specialist or other healthcare professional.

Note from the authors:

> The purpose of this book is to ensure you have all the information you need so that you can advocate for yourself and find the best care, as it may not always be offered as standard to mothers. Some healthcare systems are better than others, and some cultures prioritize maternal health and postpartum recovery more than others, but we believe that everyone should have access to enough information to make informed choices about their recovery.

> As you read through the book, we hope you will feel able to plan for a positive birth experience and for your confidence to grow in your postpartum body. While Caesarean birth does come with some challenges, it can also be a wonderful experience, and with the right advice and support the recovery is made so much easier. We're extremely proud to have written this book and so grateful for the willingness and enthusiasm of the C-section families and other postpartum experts who have contributed and expressed their desire to support other parents. We hope our book will help you, and many more women, to feel great and thrive in motherhood after a C-section birth.

> Love Hannah and Emma xx

1

Different types of C-sections

If you have a Caesarean birth you will either have an elective (planned) C-section, or an emergency Caesarean (when your vaginal birth results in a C-section birth).

What is an elective C-section?

An elective C-section means that your C-section is planned and scheduled before you go into labour. The date of your operation is usually before your due date to avoid you going into labour before, but depending on your reason for having this type of birth, you may be able to choose the date or your doctor may recommend when they feel it's best to book it in.

Why might you have an elective C-section?

There are a number of reasons you may need an elective C-section, such as:

- You have placenta previa. This is when your placenta is covering your cervix, blocking the baby's way out. Vaginal birth would most likely cause severe bleeding and be very dangerous.
- You have other health issues that mean a C-section is the safest option for you. This may include things like HIV or genital herpes that could be passed on to your baby via a vaginal birth, diabetes or pre-eclampsia (high blood pressure).*
- Multiples – if you're having twins, triplets or more, it may be advised that you have a C-section. This is not always the case with twins, but very likely if you're having more babies.
- Your baby is in a position which makes vaginal birth more difficult or impossible, such as if the baby is in a breech presentation (bottom first).

*Although these issues may mean a C-section is advised, it doesn't mean it's your only option. Women with active genital herpes are often advised to take antivirals from 36 weeks pregnant and to plan for a vaginal birth. Well-controlled diabetes in pregnant women often means they have normal-sized babies.

- If you've had previous C-sections or other surgeries to your womb. Research shows that the risk of complications in pregnancy and future births does rise with multiple C-sections, and this may influence the advice or preferences of your birth team. However, many women do go on to have a successful VBAC (Vaginal Birth After a C-section) and you should be supported to have these conversations with your birth team if it is your wish.

Not all these concerns mean that a Caesarean is the only option, so speak with your medical provider to discuss all your options. Don't be afraid to advocate for yourself, do your research and request another medical provider if you feel you're not being heard.

Can you still have an elective C-section even if you don't fit any of these criteria?

Yes, it's your body and you can choose how you want to birth your baby. You will need to chat to your doctor about this and they will want to know your reasons, to make sure it's the right birth choice for you.

Go in prepared: have a list ready of your reasons for wanting a C-section and your feelings around this. You may find that after chatting it through you change your mind or, if it's fear of birth that's brought you to this decision, that you may be referred to speak to a birth counsellor.

A C-section is major surgery that will leave you with scar tissue for the rest of your life, so it is not a decision that should be made lightly, but you should never feel forced into a choice that isn't right for you. If you feel like you're not being listened to or supported, request to speak to another medical provider.

Questions you may want to ask your medical provider when planning a C-section

- Why do I need to have a C-section? Are there any alternatives?
- Will having a C-section cause any problems for me or my baby?
- If it's due to a 'large baby', why do they believe your baby is large and how accurate is this measurement?

- It's better for your baby to be born as close to term as possible, so find out if there's a problem with you or your baby's health that makes it necessary for them to be born prior to 39 weeks. Is it safe/ possible to move your date any closer to term?
- Is it possible to have a vaginal birth with future pregnancies?
- If you are prone to raised or keloid scars, make the surgeon aware and ask if they have any suggestions about what they may be able to do to limit this.

What is an emergency C-section?

An emergency C-section is often not as drastic or immediate as it sounds, and can refer to any Caesarean section that has not been previously planned but has become the safest option for both you and baby.

Why might you have an emergency C-section?

Reasons for why your birth may result in an emergency C-section include:

- Any of the above reasons for having an elective C-section, such as breech positioning or placenta previa having been discovered after you went into labour.
- Going into labour before your scheduled elective C-section date.
- Your baby being in foetal distress but the labour hasn't progressed enough to have a forceps or ventouse delivery.
- Your labour is not progressing as expected, your contractions aren't effective or your cervix hasn't opened enough.
- Unexpected complications such as a cord prolapse (where the cord slips out before the baby) or placental abruption (a serious condition in which the placenta separates from the wall of the uterus before birth).
- Your baby's head is deemed too big for your pelvis or baby is in the wrong position.
- You develop a serious condition like severe pre-eclampsia (high blood pressure) or heart disease.
- Heavy bleeding from your vagina.
- A failed induction – you have been induced but labour doesn't begin.
- A failed assisted delivery – forceps or ventouse have been tried but failed to deliver your baby.

Different types of emergency C-section

The reason you need an emergency C-section and the level of urgency will determine what type of C-section your birth is classified as.

A Category 3 C-section is when there's no immediate danger to either you or baby so there isn't a pressing deadline. A scenario for this may be that you are scheduled for an elective C-section, but your waters have broken or labour has begun.

A Category 2 C-section is more urgent and usually aims to get your baby born within 90 minutes of the decision. This might be necessary if there are signs that either you or your baby are not doing well during the labour process. It could be due to a range of issues, such as severe pre-eclampsia or if labour isn't progressing as expected and there are signs of distress in your baby.

A Category 1 C-section is the most urgent type of emergency C-section and is often referred to as a 'Crash' C-section. This is when your baby needs to be born immediately, ideally within 30 minutes of the decision. This extreme urgency could be due to several reasons, such as your baby showing signs of significant distress, heavy vaginal bleeding, or a prolapsed umbilical cord.

Each category is designed to ensure the safety and well-being of both mother and baby, responding appropriately to the urgency of the situation.

Questions to ask if you're told you need an emergency C-section

We recommend highlighting this section of the book, or putting it somewhere for your partner to access if necessary and advocate for you.

- Am I or my baby in immediate distress?
- If there are signs of foetal distress what are they?
- Do I have any other options other than a C-section?
- Can we delay the decision to have a C-section?

Risks of having a Caesarean

C-sections are a widely practised and on the whole safe method of childbirth, however, as with any surgical procedure, there are associated risks. These risks will vary depending on whether the C-section is planned or an emergency, and your general health will play a role too. Before the procedure, your healthcare team will discuss the potential risks and benefits to ensure you have all the necessary information. But if you're thinking of planning a C-section it's important to be aware of the risks when making your decision.

Risks to the mother

- Wound infection: It's not uncommon to get an infection in the wound after birth. Signs of this include: Redness, swelling, oozing or discomfort at the wound site (we go into more detail on this in a later chapter). The sooner these infections are caught the better, but they often clear up with antibiotics.
- Infection in the womb lining: Things to look out for are: Fever, abdominal pain, unusual discharge, or heavy bleeding. While common, these infections can be managed with appropriate medical care.
- Excessive bleeding: This is less common and may require additional medical intervention, such as a blood transfusion or further surgery. This can happen on the operating table or post-surgery, but you will be closely monitored after birth.
- Reactions to the anaesthetic: It is possible to have a reaction to any type of anaesthetic.
- Deep vein thrombosis (DVT): This rare condition involves a blood clot in the leg and needs careful postoperative care. Your medical team will help prevent this through the use of compression socks during and after surgery, blood thinning injections post-birth and getting you up and moving regularly post-birth.
- Bladder or bowel damage: Also rare, but can be treated with additional medical procedures.

Women are often given antibiotics before a C-section to help limit the chance of infection.

Risks to the baby

- Minor skin cuts: Occasionally, the baby may sustain a small cut during the procedure. These cuts are usually minor and heal quickly.
- Breathing difficulties: This is more common in babies born before 39 weeks and generally improves within a few days. Your baby will be closely monitored during this time.

If you notice any concerns about your baby's breathing after leaving the hospital, seek medical advice immediately.

Vaginal birth after Caesarean (VBAC)

Just because you have had a C-section, this doesn't necessarily mean that future pregnancies have to also be born via C-section. Some women may be advised to have another Caesarean with subsequent pregnancies, but this depends on whether a C-section is still, or is now the safest option for them and their baby.

For most women, the possibility of a vaginal birth after a Caesarean (VBAC) is a common and safe option. In fact, a significant number of women who have had a C-section go on to have a vaginal delivery in their subsequent pregnancies.

The advantages are:

- Having a VBAC involves no surgery and therefore less potential for complications during surgery.
- You're likely to be in hospital for less time and recover and be back to 'normal' activities quicker, too.

For some women, experiencing vaginal childbirth is also important to them and wanting to have a large family may also influence your decision, as it isn't advised to have more than three C-sections due to the increased risk of uterine and placental problems.

Things that need to be considered before making this decision:

- Health considerations: Your overall health, the health of your baby, and the reasons for your initial C-section play a crucial role in determining whether a VBAC is a suitable option (see above for possible reasons for a planned C-section).
- How long ago your previous C-section was: If your pregnancy is less than 18 months from your previous one, it's unlikely you will

be offered a VBAC. The risk of uterine rupture is higher due to the scar tissue on your uterus not having yet matured to be at optimum strength.

- Type of uterine incision: The type of incision made in your previous C-section affects the decision. Most C-sections are performed with a low horizontal cut along your bikini line. However, vertical cuts pose a higher risk of uterine rupture, so it's unlikely a VBAC will be advised in this case.
- Other surgeries to your uterus: multiple other surgeries to your uterus such as fibroid removal may mean a VBAC isn't recommended.
- Multiple C-sections: If you've had more than two C-sections it's likely you won't be offered a VBAC for subsequent pregnancies.
- Hospital policies and resources: Some hospitals may not have the necessary resources to safely conduct a VBAC, especially if an emergency arises.

Risks of a VBAC – there are less complications associated with successful vaginal births after a C-section compared to having a planned C-section, however when labour is unsuccessful after a previous C-section, there is potential for greater complications such as uterine rupture. Although this is rare, it's a serious life threatening emergency where the scar on your uterus from your previous C-section splits open. In this instance a Category 1 (see above) C-section would be performed and potentially a hysterectomy (where your uterus is removed).

How is labour different with a VBAC?

Your birth choice is yours and many women have successfully had a VBAC at home or with minimal intervention. However, what is likely to be advised to you by your medical team, is that you have a VBAC in hospital in case an emergency C-section is needed. It is also often recommended to have extra monitoring during labour, meaning the baby's heartbeat is continuously monitored to make sure everything is progressing well and that the baby isn't in any distress, which could indicate you may need another C-section. While being monitored, it does mean you are unable to have a water birth or able to labour in the water.

You can have an epidural if you want to, and this can be used as the anaesthetic if your labour does turn into a C-section birth.

Induction with a VBAC

Induction with a VBAC is not usually recommended as it increases the risk of the scar on your uterus from your previous C-section rupturing by two to three times when compared to labour starting by itself. Uterine rupture is a medical emergency but it is still rare, and only happens to one to two women in every 100. Induced VBACs also have a lower success rate of 67 in 100.[3] This means that if you were overdue with your pregnancy you are likely to be recommended that the best option for you would be to have a repeat C-section.

But as we've said previously, it's your body, your choice. Going to the hospital prepared, having done your research and voiced any questions and concerns to your medical team prior to delivery, will give you the confidence to make an informed choice about what is best for you and your baby.

Home birth after a C-section

Although you are likely to be advised against having an HBAC (home birth after a C-section) you can (always) choose the option that is right for you. One study found that:[4]

- Women who planned an HBAC compared to a VBAC in a hospital setting had a significantly increased chance of vaginal birth.
- In both home and hospital settings, the chances of negative outcomes were low, but still worth considering.
- The chances of having to be transferred from home to hospital during birth are high in women planning an HBAC, at 37 per cent and with second babies 57 per cent.

It's important to discuss any concerns or future pregnancy plans with your healthcare provider for tailored advice. You will be offered a VBAC appointment during your third trimester, so go prepared with your questions.

We've made a list here to get you started:

Questions to ask your healthcare provider when considering a VBAC

- Does the reason for my previous C-section in any way indicate that I need another C-section?
- Is there anything about my current pregnancy that affects my decision?
- What are my risks when having a VBAC compared to a planned C-section?
- What are my risks of having an HBAC compared to a VBAC or planned C-section?

My birth story: Liz

I have had two C-sections, one emergency and one elective. Both amazing, both very different.

With my first pregnancy, I really wanted a totally natural birth, as many women do. We attended many antenatal courses, including 'parent school', about looking after your newborn, antenatal yoga, and one-to-one hypnobirthing. There was a focus on how your body is designed to birth, and intervention isn't good for this process. I was very comfortable and focused on this way of thinking.

Unfortunately, my body had other ideas. At around 30 weeks, my blood pressure started to rise, and so I was closely monitored. A few weeks later, it was clear I had developed pre-eclampsia. Even though the doctors advised me to have an early induction, I held strong until my due date. But by this point, there was a risk to both me and the baby, so I went to the hospital on my due date to be induced.

Starting with a hormonal pessary, labour was initiated. I used the hypnobirthing techniques that I had learned, but there was no progress. Hours passed, and I was given a second pessary. At this point, the wonderful midwifery team covered all the medical equipment with sheets and put a notice on the door to give us time and space to try to get a natural birth in motion. But it was not to be.

My blood pressure was now at a critical level, and the oral medication was not having any effect. So, I was put on a drip, which was by far the worst feeling of the whole intervention. The contractions continued, but unfortunately, I had only dilated by 4 cm. I had refused to have my waters broken by the consultant who had arrived with the needle but had not consulted me, so I sent her away.

I had lost track of time, but after going in on Wednesday morning, it was now some point on Friday, and it was time to decide on the next step. Having been given information about the oxytocin drip (another part of the induction process), the likely increase in pain, and the fact I was totally exhausted, I agreed to have an epidural.

I was given the epidural and then the oxytocin drip. I could feel the 'banging' sensation of the strong contractions, but overall, I felt calmer. Unfortunately, at this point, the strong squeeze of the contractions was affecting our baby's heart rate, and we were advised the safest way forward was to birth via Caesarean section. I quickly agreed, as by this point we were just thinking about the safety of our baby.

I was prepped for surgery and taken into the theatre. I thought 'what a wonderful place' (I know this seems a strange thing to say). There was an amazing all-female team working in synchrony. The whole experience felt serene. Though I am sure it may not have been as calm as I felt (as it was an emergency), I knew I was in good hands. At 9.32 p.m. on 1 December, 60 hours after arriving at the hospital, we saw our little girl. She was checked over, held by my husband, and then passed to me for our skin-to-skin time.

With my second pregnancy, I was closely monitored, and spent a lot of time talking to my midwife about birth choices. I still had a longing for a natural birth, but there were so many unknowns, and a risk of intervention that could lead me down the same path as the first time. In the end, my midwife asked a very straightforward question: 'Disregarding all other factors, what do you really want for this birth?' and the answer was calmness and control over the situation. Therefore, an elective C-section was my heart's choice. It had been the best part of the first birth, and I knew what to expect. Although it is abdominal surgery, I was reassured by my midwife that it is very safe.

It is exciting and strange to know exactly when your baby is going to be born. There are still nerves, but with elective surgery, there are some lovely choices such as not cutting the cord immediately and skin-to-skin. You can still make a birth plan, and the baby will be birthed slowly, allowing time for their adjustment, closer to a vaginal birth. I felt safe and supported; this was the right route for me and our baby.

We were first on the list the day of the birth, and my blood pressure was behaving, so everything was good to go. As with all surgery, you cannot eat before, so I was happy; we were first in. They administered the spinal to numb my body, and then I was taken into surgery. The team talked me through everything, and then my little boy was handed to me for skin-to-skin time.

After the surgery, I was taken down to the maternity ward and saw some familiar faces from three years previously. The team encouraged me to get on my feet as soon as I felt comfortable. I had my catheter and cannula removed that night. I was discharged the following day, feeling proud and happy with the choices we had made. There was still quite a long recovery, my husband had to administer anticoagulant injections for a number of days, and in hindsight I wish I had stayed in one extra night.

The recovery from both of my births went well, ensuring I was mobile and going to the loo as soon as possible. The wound is covered initially with a clear dressing and the midwife comes to check it is all healing well. The first time I had a proper look I was surprised how quickly the skin bonds to itself. There are many strange feelings, like the first shower and the first time you cough or sneeze is definitely memorable! The main thing I remember being told was to keep moving and walking.

I had read about looking after my scar, and once it was healed over, to massage it, helping the healing process and blood flow. I did this to some extent (and only very lightly) and at the time felt it had healed well. The thing I hadn't considered the second time was that the surgery would be in the same place and this may well change the amount of scar tissue or how it healed.

After my second C-section the scar healed well in general but it definitely felt and looked different. One side (the left, my preferred sleeping side) was smooth and pale but the right-hand side was lumpier and darker and the whole scar was tight with an overhang of flesh. The appearance didn't really bother me but the sensation became more uncomfortable and I was having much worse ovulation pain.

The discomfort got to the point I was constantly aware of the scar and so sought help; this came in the form of Hannah West. She is brilliant at explaining about the healing process of all the layers of the body that are affected by the surgery. And though I had been lightly massaging the exterior I wasn't addressing the scar tissue further down. I had a few sessions with Hannah along with homework of daily self-massage which became (and often still is) a part of a relaxing bedtime routine. It made such a difference, my scar improved visibly, the tightness and overhang had gone and, more importantly for me, I have no physical awareness of it. I wish there had been more information provided about how to look after your healing scar and that there is help out there if you need it.

2

How to prepare for a C-section

If you're having a planned C-section there's lots you can do to prepare for the operation. To make sure you're in the right place physically and mentally, to have the best possible experience and to be able to recover well. But even if you're planning a vaginal birth, one in four births in the UK[1] or one in three in the USA[5] are now via C-section so it's really beneficial to be prepared for any eventuality. It can be challenging to learn these things post-birth when you're exhausted, recovering and caring for a new baby.

Finding out what's involved during the surgery, what to expect whilst you're in hospital and from your recovery can help you feel more in control and more prepared. We've included lots of information on all this in other chapters within this book.

What you can do for your body pre-operation

Not all these things are possible when you're heavily pregnant, uncomfortable and needing to get up to pee a hundred times in the night. But even small changes can make a big difference to how well your body recovers from surgery.

- Try to focus on daily movement, even ten minutes of gentle yoga or walking counts.
- Good nutrition pre-op as well as plenty of water and appropriate supplements can help put your body in a great place for birth and recovery.
- Sleep – if you're not sleeping well, can you go to bed earlier or take a nap in the day? Even lying still on the bed for 15 minutes is a rest, and will help your body be in a better place for birth. Try to think of it as adding some savings to your bank of energy as you'll likely be depleted post-birth.
- Start your pelvic floor exercises in pregnancy. If you've read Chapter 15 already, you'll know that the weight of pregnancy on your pelvic

floor muscles is the main cause of pelvic floor problems post-birth so it doesn't matter how you birth your baby, you still need to focus on these, and a strong pelvic floor pre-birth will improve your recovery after. It's also easier for you to connect with those muscles after delivery when you may be tired or sore if you've been practising them regularly before.

- Mental preparation – if you're feeling anxious or nervous, practising meditation, mindfulness or journaling, can really help you to process your thoughts or fears and identify ways to help manage your emotions during your birth. Often parents describe feeling 'out of control' during a birth, particularly if that includes being in a surgical theatre, as the medical team sometimes has to work quickly. It's often that loss of control or fear of the unknown that triggers traumatic or negative feelings, or physical responses such as tensing your muscles or the nervous system being in 'fight-or-flight' mode. Having a plan ahead of time that you and your partner can focus on together gives you back some control and can stop you from spiralling. Lots of people have very positive experiences with a C-section birth, and we've included a number of real life birth stories within this book. But the common factors are usually to do with making the environment feel calm or safe, or feeling properly informed about what's happening. These are things you can do for yourself, with some preparation.

- Hypnobirthing is also a really beneficial practice for C-section births as well as vaginal births to help you cope.

- Get your scar recovery products ready for post-birth. You can wear compression underwear as soon as you feel ready, so you may want to bring these to the hospital with you. Having your scar oils and silicone strips ready for you at home will save you having to worry about this after birth. For more information see Chapter 11 on C-section recovery products.

- It's worth planning a couple of outfits for a hospital stay and what you'll wear to come home in, as you'll want loose, light layers and underwear that sits above your scar: avoid any waistbands that would press or rub over your wound site. Consider whether you plan to breastfeed; if you end up staying in hospital for a few days you'll also want to choose something you can unbutton or easily move to feed or even just for skin-to-skin contact.

- Read Chapter 7 on early scar and wound care. Often, little information is given about this from the hospital. Good wound care from day one can prevent infection, speed up the healing process of your scar, and improve the outcome and resulting symptoms. Knowing this pre-operation can help you give your wound the best possible outcome, as can knowing how to spot any warning signs of an infection early on.
- Colostrum harvesting – from 36 weeks pregnant you can collect your colostrum, the first milk your body makes. It contains antibodies to protect your baby from infection, and helps their immune and digestive systems to develop, protecting them from allergies. It also helps to reduce the chances of jaundice by encouraging your baby to open their bowels to pass their first poo and clear meconium from the digestive tract. Studies have shown that having a C-section may delay the start of mature milk production. Having an anaesthetic may also make your baby drowsy at first, potentially affecting their ability to feed initially. Your levels of pain, your emotions, and if your baby needs to go into intensive care also all have the potential to affect your ability to breastfeed at the start. Not only will collecting your colostrum pre-birth mean that you have some of this liquid gold ready to give to your baby in these instances, but it will also encourage your milk to come in sooner. Make sure you speak to your midwife or medical provider before beginning this, and seek their support if you're finding your feeding journey difficult.
- Hair removal – please speak to your medical team beforehand. Some will ask you to remove excess hair if they feel it will be in the way. It should be done with clippers rather than a razor as a razor may cause small skin breaks and increase the chances of skin infection.

If you only do one thing before your C-section...

Prepare others and ask for help. We know not everyone has a big support system in place, but asking for help pre-birth can take the pressure off you. Let whoever you live with know that you will need to rest in order to recover; can they put things in place to make that happen? Can a friend collect any older children you have from school/nursery for a couple of weeks? If you have a toddler or older children have a chat with them, let them know you won't be able to lift them for a while and you need their help. Setting up some play or activity and snack stations in the rooms you're likely to spend the most time in can be a good idea to keep other children happy while you're resting or feeding. At the bare minimum make it known you won't be cooking and cleaning for a couple of weeks!

Home preparation before your C-section

Getting your home ready for when you come back from hospital after the birth can make the world of difference in enabling you to rest and recover better.

- Meal preparation – batch cooking lots of protein-rich, easy-to-reheat and frozen meals means you won't have to worry about cooking anything for a while when you first get home. It will also ensure that you can eat nutritious, healing meals, which will speed up your recovery. Take a look at Chapter 8 on nutrition for ideas.
- You could also request that, rather than presents for the new baby, friends and family bring round meals for you or buy you a meal subscription service for a few weeks.
- Cleaning – if you know this is something that will bother you, ask for a partner or people who share your home to take this on for a couple of weeks in order to permit you to rest. Another great new baby present or investment would be for someone to pay for a cleaner for a few weeks so you're not going to be straining your new scar pushing the hoover, leaning over toilets and carrying heavy baskets of clothes. Or if people are coming round to visit, ask them to help.
- Get everything you need for you and baby in one place so that, if you're planning on hanging out in your bedroom for the first couple of weeks (which would be a great idea), you don't need to be going up and down the stairs all day. Make sure you have a large water bottle for yourself, a flask you or others can fill full of tea/coffee, snacks, plenty of painkillers and your schedule for taking them, maternity sanitary pads, a changing mat for baby, a place for them to sleep downstairs to avoid carrying a bassinet upstairs and downstairs and plenty of nappies and

a few changes of clothes. Fill a caddy up with all these things for if you need to move to a different room.

- It can be really challenging to get out of bed at first; it may be painful to move or your core may feel very weak, making it difficult to sit up from bed as usual. Tying a belt to the end of your bed, or a door handle if your bed is close enough that you can use to help pull yourself upright can be a real game-changer, especially if you may not have someone around to help you all the time.
- Poop stool – constipation and fear of going to the toilet post-birth can make it hard to go. By elevating your feet on to a stool in front of the toilet, your colon will be in the best position to pass a bowel movement. You can buy stools specifically for this but even an upturned bucket will do the trick.

Hospital preparation before your C-section

There are a number of items that you can add to your hospital bag that will especially help if you have a C-section. We've created a list you can download and tick off here:

Hospital bag

https://subscribepage.io/SA24QS

- Make a playlist – even if you're having an unplanned C-section it's likely in most cases you will be able to play your own music in theatre. Preparing a list of songs that are going to make you feel more relaxed and in control can really help.
- Your birth plan. These are some things you may want to consider/discuss pre-birth with your medical provider if you are having a C-section or in case you end up having a C-section.

- Drape lowering – do you want to be able to see your baby being born/is this something the hospital offers?
- Cord cutting – does your partner want to be able to do this, does the hospital allow it?
- Delayed clamping (this can help prevent your baby from getting anaemia and increase the transfer of stem cells) – is this something you want to have, how long would you like to leave it and is it something the hospital can facilitate?
- Skin-to-skin contact with your baby after birth is known to expose babies to the beneficial microbiomes on the mother's skin. If your baby is well, you can request skin-to-skin straight away without them being weighed so you may want to add this to your written birth plan so the team is aware of your wishes.
- Vaginal seeding – this practice involves taking a swab from your vagina shortly after giving birth via C-section and wiping it over babies mouth, nose, skin, face and eyes in the hope that the beneficial bacteria the baby would have been exposed to during a vaginal birth will boost the baby's gut bacteria and reduce the risk of allergies, immune disorders and asthma. Further research is required in this field and it has not yet been approved for practice in the UK or USA, so we'd recommend speaking with your midwife or medical provider in advance to ask for their opinion.
- Breastfeeding will also help to support a healthy microbiome, so this is something you may wish to consider when making feeding choices.
- Make sure you follow the guidelines from your surgeon on eating and drinking guidelines the night before. You will likely be able to eat normally the night before and be able to continue to drink water until some point in the morning. This will depend on what time your operation is booked for, and you will be told the exact time to stop at your pre-operation appointment that you will have sometime in the week before your C-section. Be prepared to feel hungry on the day, and know that you may have to wait longer than expected if an emergency C-section case takes priority.

Every medical team will likely have their own lists of accepted practices, but discussing your preferences in advance makes it more likely that you'll have the experience you want.

Other things to consider

Keloid scars

If you are prone to keloid scarring or have a family history of keloid scars, if possible talk to your surgeon beforehand to see if they have any solutions to help prevent and reduce the formation of this scar type.

It's advisable to use compression underwear or garments over this scar type as soon as possible to prevent the excessive production of collagen that causes it, so you may want to pack yours in your hospital bag. Make sure you have silicone dressings ready at home for the early days and, once your wound is closed over, your reusable silicone strip to continue the care.

We cover the different types of scars in Chapter 22.

Plus-size women

If your tummy folds over your incision site, your wound is likely to take longer to heal as air is not easily able to get to it. We would recommend talking to your surgeon about a pico dressing. We have included lots of other tips to help with C-section overhang in Chapter 7 on early scar care; Chapter 23 is a whole chapter devoted to C-section overhang.

If you are diabetic

If you are diabetic it's really important your blood sugar is carefully monitored and well controlled. High blood sugar levels can increase the risk of infection at the wound site. The fatigue and exertion of birth can make it harder to control your blood sugar levels for a while, hence why you'll be monitored closely. This may impact how long you are advised to stay in hospital for after your birth. Because diabetes may mean your wound is slower to heal, the following advice is particularly important for you:

- Getting adequate rest and sleep to give your body the best chance to heal effectively.
- Eating nutritious meals.
- Taking time out for self-care to help manage your stress and energy levels.

- Keep regular appointments with your doctor or healthcare provider to check blood sugar and insulin levels regularly.
- When you have recovered well enough, introduce regular movement and exercise as part of your general management of your condition.

This advice can also apply if you've been diagnosed with gestational diabetes in pregnancy. Usually this is a temporary diagnosis and will resolve after birth, but it can take up to 6–12 weeks to disappear, so you should be monitored and supported by your medical team during the postpartum phase.

Reading this information in advance should help you to create a birth plan that addresses the things that are important to you. Your birth team should be supportive of your choices and provide you with relevant information to support any clinical decisions, and you are entitled to ask questions if you're not happy with or sure about any decisions. Having some control over the birth experience for both you and your birth partner can often make the experience much more enjoyable and positively impact your emotional and physical wellbeing after.

My birth story: Gabriella

I had a very positive experience!

I always knew I was terrified of giving birth, but until I fell pregnant I didn't realize how severe this fear was. I was assigned a wonderful midwife who picked up on my fear at my 10-week appointment and referred me to the NHS perinatal mental health services, who were incredible. I did do a little bit of hypnobirthing preparation just in case, but after multiple sessions it was agreed I would chat to an obstetrician to discuss an elective C-section. My obstetrician was also wonderful, and once a date was set I finally relaxed!

We got to the hospital at 8 a.m. on the day of the C-section. The anaesthetist and surgeon introduced themselves in the morning, and my wonderful midwife who had looked after me during my whole pregnancy came in on her day off to wish me good luck. Because I was the lowest priority I didn't end up in theatre until 2 p.m. The wait at the hospital was quite stressful, but we set up the laptop and watched some reality TV, and occasionally my partner would advise me to do some hypnobirthing 'upbreathing' to help with my nerves.

Around 2 p.m. we moved into theatre – everyone was super friendly. They popped on our playlist (which my partner had made the night before!) and prepped me for the spinal injection. I did unfortunately have a bit of a nervous breakdown at this point. I was sobbing too hard for the anaesthetist to safely administer the spinal but I again used some hypnobirthing up-breathing (coached by my partner!) to get through this.

Once the injection was over I felt a tingly sensation all over – my blood pressure did unfortunately plummet and this was a truly awful feeling – I felt incredibly nauseous and like I was going to pass out but the anaesthetist quickly sorted this. Within the next five to ten minutes my baby was born! It was honestly the most surreal and incredible moment when they dropped the curtain to show her to us. The midwife took some incredible photos, and she was co-incidentally born to the song we had chosen for our first dance at our wedding (planned for six months after her birth). So special. She came out perfect, screaming and crying and had no issues whatsoever. She was handed to me and lay on my chest for the rest of the operation.

It took around 40 minutes to suture me up – I am a vet so I had a lovely chat with everyone about the differences between C-sections in animals versus in people. And everyone approved very much of my partner's playlist and said we could come back for another C-section any time (no thank you!).

I was wheeled through to recovery and genuinely felt like a new woman – all my anxieties instantly gone. I was looked after with such care and compassion that night – the nurses made sure my bedsheets were kept clean, they frequently checked I had enough pain relief on board and removed my urinary catheter around 2 a.m. I was discharged exactly 24 hours after the operation, after they had checked my wound and performed some final checks on our baby.

I had a wonderful postpartum experience. Luckily, breastfeeding was fine, my baby latched well and my milk came in 48 hours after she was born. I didn't have any baby blues or any other mental health issues going forward, and was discharged from perinatal mental health services after four weeks once they were satisfied I was fine.

The recovery was very painful, but I was looked after so well and it was a small price to pay for such a positive experience. I followed The 360 Mama recovery programme and now at four months postpartum I have no overhang and only a slightly red scar. The NHS really is wonderful, and I feel so lucky to have been looked after so incredibly well throughout my whole journey.

3

Hypnobirthing for a Caesarean birth

Taking ownership of your birth experience and introducing things that help you to feel calm, happy and positive before, during and after the birth is one of the most effective ways to influence how your birth goes. Ultimately birth is often unpredictable, so where possible it's a good idea to include things in your birth plan you know you can control, which can be applied in any circumstance. This is why we've asked Laura Batten, a hypnobirthing instructor and birth doula to offer some guidance about using hypnobirthing techniques for a Caesarean birth. We love how she also includes the ways in which hypnobirthing can be beneficial for your pregnancy and how to use the skills for coping in parenthood long after your birth, too – so whatever stage you're at, there's something useful for you in this chapter.

I've always thought 'hypnobirthing' has the wrong name. It conjures up ideas of being hypnotized, and certainly not something you need in a Caesarean birth. So, let's explore what hypnobirthing really is, and how it's applicable, relevant and empowering to *all* births.

Hypnobirthing is a way to calm and reframe your inner thoughts, which sit in your subconscious mind. Your feelings and emotions directly impact your behaviours, attitudes, beliefs and actions, so by changing the story you tell yourself you're able to impact how your mind and body reacts. In scientific terms, this reframing to create positive neural pathways is called neuroplasticity.

Simply put, hypnobirthing is about a mind–body connection – the psychology of birth (what's happening in your mind), along with the physiology (what's happening in your body). Hypnobirthing techniques can help you feel confident and calm, and help you have a more connected experience of pregnancy, birth and your postnatal period. Hypnobirthing is a way to regain control, build resilience and create a positive mindset towards a birth you can be fully involved in.

Hopefully, on this understanding, you can see how hypnobirthing techniques can help anyone, and can help you plan for a more connected experience as you approach your Caesarean birth.

I work as a birth doula and have supported parents during both planned and unplanned Caesarean births. But we don't just turn up on the day and start using a bit of breathing to get through the birth; there's so much intention, learning and un-learning that begins as early in pregnancy as you'd like. So, how can hypnobirthing be used in planning for a Caesarean birth (whether it's elective or emergency), and what skills can you learn?

- **Breathwork**: Utilize your breath to help you stay calm, and out of your fight/flight nervous system.
- **Visualization**: Strengthen your mind–body connection using specific and personalized visualization methods to connect with baby and yourself.
- **Reframing**: Work on the story you tell yourself and choose to change the narrative through practices like positive affirmations and fear release.
- **Environment preparation**: Focus on which senses and what sensory stimulation around you will help you feel grounded and manage your feelings around birth and postpartum.
- **Hormonal production**: Learn how your hormones are produced and how they can help/hinder you, and specifically how a Caesarean birth impacts your hormones.
- **Speaking up**: Become confident and empowered to make requests and advocate for yourself, with birth choices that feel right for you.
- **Peace and connection**: Develop a sense of peace and contentment about your decisions, balance your emotions during pregnancy, and look forward to your connected experience of birth.

Hopefully you can see how hypnobirthing isn't just for contractions! It's also not about glossing over challenges – quite the opposite. It's identifying challenges, validating your feelings around them, and finding techniques to help you not just manage, but feel proud about and even enjoy moving through them. These are skills for life!

Hypnobirthing is for the pregnancy too, not just the birth

Practising hypnobirthing techniques during pregnancy can have a wealth of positive impacts on your mind and growing body; here are a few:

- A more regulated nervous system, practising being in your 'calm and content' mode.
- The ability to move out of flight-or-flight mode to help adrenaline subside.
- Increased connection with your mind, body and baby.
- Decreased feelings of overwhelm or lack of control.
- Being more emotionally grounded and able to look forward to birth.
- Reassurance that however you birth you have useful skills – even if your labour leads to an emergency Caesarean birth.

Hypnobirthing during pregnancy can help build confidence, release fear, help you focus on what you can control, and meaningfully change how your subconscious brain is processing everything.

I'd highly recommend taking a bespoke Caesarean birth preparation course that includes hypnobirthing and postnatal preparation. I teach my Mindful Natal® Caesarean course through The Mindful Birth Group, but there are other providers and teachers who also focus on this birth choice. Not all courses are created equally though, so be sure to talk to your potential teacher about their approach and what they cover, and make sure it aligns with what you want to achieve. I'd recommend choosing a course that also covers 'unexpected turns', because some planned Caesarean babies decide to start making their way earthside before the elected date! In that scenario, it's going to be comforting to know that if you chose to go ahead with a vaginal birth (or if baby was coming so quickly that you didn't have time to decide otherwise!) then you have the skills you need to help you.

One of the many reasons why hypnobirthing practices are so helpful when planning a Caesarean birth, is that they can change how you feel about the birth, *during* your pregnancy. The time spent preparing is valuable.

Using an analogy of planning for a big holiday a few months away, you could:

- Use reputable resources to find out what it's really like where you're going.
- Pour over amazing photos and videos of your destination.
- Build your own itinerary; not someone else's.
- Pack your favourite things for comfort and fun.
- Learn a skill that will enhance your trip – like learning some words in a new language.

If you do it this way, you get the pleasure in the planning; you feel excited about your decisions knowing the trip will be unique to you and so much more enjoyable for it.

Or otherwise, you could:

- Just not think about it at all, and deal with it when the day comes.
- Look at only negative reviews.
- Leave your belongings at home and rely on the hotel's provision.
- Leave everything to a professional travel agent with no input of your own on your likes and dislikes.
- Assume that once you arrive everyone will speak your language.

If you do it this way, it's unlikely that you'll have an experience that is personal to you, or one you're hugely invested in. In short: it won't be yours, and it may not be just right for you.

Big Holiday vs Giving Birth; it's not a watertight analogy, but hopefully you see where I'm going with it! I really encourage you to adopt the mindset that learning these skills is an investment for your pregnancy and postnatal experience, as much as it is for your birth.

Your senses

We're all familiar with our five senses – sight, hearing, touch, smell and taste. But it's hotly debated about how many additional senses we have (some say up to 21!), and I believe the lesser-known senses are a real key to preparing for a Caesarean birth. Here are three under-the-radar senses that I think are important to value during a Caesarean birth.

- **Proprioception** – *the sense and perception of body awareness*. What can you feel happening in your body during your time in theatre? How might that make you feel? The concept of not being able to feel your body when it's anaesthetised may be completely new to you, and worth being prepared for from someone who knows the process.

- **Chemical senses** – *such as the sense for hunger, water or air.* Planned Caesarean births require nil-by-mouth from the morning of Birth Day, so it's important to consider how your body and mind may feel under those conditions. Not being able to meet those basic needs – including after birth while you slowly reintroduce them – is worth mentally preparing for and having tools up your sleeve to manage.
- **Mental senses** – *pain (external or internal), mental or spiritual distress, sense of self.* There may be a reason that your mental senses are heightened in the lead up to birth, depending on your reasons and feelings about the decision to birth abdominally. How can you practise supporting your mind in times of stress, and how can your birth partner hold that space for you?

Language and the limbic brain

You might have noticed that I use the term 'Caesarean birth' instead of C-section. There's no difference between these two events, so does it really matter what we call it? Whichever words you choose, you're not physically changing the way your baby is being born, but the use of language can hugely influence how your subconscious mind processes things, and therefore how your mind and body react to it.

I regularly do word-association exercises with my clients to prove the point that our subconscious mind really is in charge, and the phrase 'C-section' generally evokes the following responses for them: surgery, medical, clinical, process, out of control. It might be worth noting down for yourself the words it brings up for you personally? When I then ask about the phrase 'Caesarean birth' (or abdominal birth) and what it evokes, the responses are generally 'more like a birth!, connected, nicer, less medical'. What words or thoughts come up for you with the switch of language? You can choose to use whatever phrases feel positive and natural to you, but it's important to spend some time noticing how these words make you feel in your body and mind. You don't just have to go with what we've culturally come to know as the go-to words. The story we tell ourselves (so, therefore, the words that we use) do have a big effect on our mindset and actions.

Hormones

Our bodies are pretty marvellous at producing hormones to coordinate different functions in our bodies. They whizz through our bloodstream to our organs, muscles and other tissues, and have a profound effect on how we feel. There are a few hormones that we're really interested in when it comes to birth and recovery, but I'd like to focus here on oxytocin and adrenaline, and how hypnobirthing and mindfulness techniques can interact with these birthing hormones.

Oxytocin is a shy hormone, and sometimes nicknamed the 'love hormone'. It comes out to play when you feel safe and loved, and has an instrumental role during physiological childbirth in the contractions of labour and in skin-to-skin contact following birth. It's important to state that less oxytocin is naturally released during an elective Caesarean birth than during a vaginal birth or an emergency Caesarean following a labour. We also know that fewer oxytocin peaks happen following an elective Caesarean birth, which does have an impact on the release of prolactin (the breastfeeding hormone). But knowledge is power, and armed with this knowledge you can feel informed and able to combat some of these discrepancies through the choices you make before, during and after your birth.

Among the important roles that oxytocin plays, the ones most relevant to a Caesarean birth are that of trust and of parent–infant bonding. Oxytocin is one of the few hormones that act in a loop-like nature. This means that the more oxytocin is released, the more your body works to release even more. So, as they say – practice makes perfect! This is your permission to start doing even more of the things you know produce oxytocin for you, so that your body starts working in this loop at every opportunity.

So, how do you produce oxytocin intentionally during pregnancy, birth and afterwards? The answer is in your sensory nerves, as when these are activated, oxytocin is released. These sensory nerves can be stimulated in many ways, but here are a few ideas:

- 'Low intensity' stimulation of the skin; stroking, reassuring physical touch or warm temperature (particularly beneficial for anti-stress). *This is really accessible during a Caesarean birth because your birth* partner or midwife will be right next to your head and able to hold your hand or have their hands on your shoulder.

- Positive, warm interaction between adults, or with animals – particularly dogs. *Whilst your canine friend won't be at your Caesarean birth, positive interaction with your birth partner or that of your care providers is important. Many of my clients find that even looking at a photo or video of their pets or family create that same warm feeling, so do consider that.*
- Receiving massage. *There may be lots of time to fill on the ward whilst you're waiting for your birth, so it's a perfect time for some massage. Postnatally, areas such as your feet, legs, hands and arms will be easily accessible and comfortable for you to have massaged.*
- During sexual intercourse and nipple stimulation. *The latter can be done before and after a Caesarean birth on the wards. The former... perhaps not in the hospital!*
- Consuming food – especially those that make you feel good! *Prepare for your postpartum with delicious, nourishing foods and snacks that are going to aid recovery.*
- Skin-to-skin contact with your baby after birth. *Baby can rest on your chest after birth, which will help with your oxytocin production – and of course all the other wonderful benefits of skin-to-skin!*

All the above – when and if they feel right for you – can induce a sense of wellbeing due to the stimulation of dopamine – another of your happy chemicals that work within your 'reward system'. When oxytocin is abundant, we see stress and anxiety wane, and even sensitivity to pain decreases in some cases. If you want to do more reading around this, it's all thanks to actions in parts of your brain call the amygdala, hypothalamic-pituitary-adrenal axis and the periaqueductal grey.

With oxytocin, endorphins and dopamine being produced, you're firmly sitting in your parasympathetic nervous system – this is your calm and content mode. This is also really important to remember for your postnatal healing to produce these feelings of wellbeing, reward and bonding.

Adrenaline is the hormone you release in response to your fight-or-flight system being activated. If you have any anxieties or fear around your Caesarean birth, you may feel the effects of adrenaline. Practising hypnobirthing during pregnancy can really help manage feelings of fear and stress and help you connect the mind and body.

Breathing techniques can help lower cortisol (the stress hormone) and increase endorphins (the body's natural pain reliever). There are a few different ways to control your breath, but essentially the idea is to slow down your breath rate.

A truly connected experience

I was once lucky enough to attend a talk by Dr Natalie Elphinstone (highly recommend a follow on Instagram). She spoke about her work in Australia and how she was striving to ensure families were seen and heard, and able to have a more connected experience with their Caesarean births. One of the many things she spoke about was the moment just before baby is born. Her standard practice is to pause at the point of entering the uterus and say to the parents 'your baby is about to be born' (or babies if it's multiples!). It might sound small, but these seven words allow parents to have that connected 'woah' moment that occurs in most vaginal births (either through feeling it yourself, or someone telling you they can see baby's head). It's things like this – that aren't widely talked about – that can really and truly make a difference to how you process your birth. You can ask your obstetrician to do what Natalie does.

How else can you make your Caesarean birth a more connected experience? Here are some ideas which I've seen work well:

- Choosing and playing your own music (it will be connected via Bluetooth to a portable speaker, often attached to the metal pole holding up the drapes near your head).
- Choosing whether or not you'd like things explained to you. Would you like to know what's happening and when? Feel free to ask questions to your anaesthetist who will be right beside you throughout. Your birth partner can also help with this; you won't be able to see much apart from the drapes and the ceiling, so having them explain what people are doing around the room can be comforting and connect you to the here and now.
- Choosing to have your ECG dots placed away from your chest, and your gown to be pulled down, to allow skin-to-skin as soon as possible after the birth.
- Choosing how low or high you'd like the drapes. It's worth reassuring you that if you choose to have the drapes lowered it does

not mean you'll be able to see into your own body – the position of your head and bump (and what remains of the drapes) just means you'd be able to more easily see baby coming out.

- Birth partner support. Reassuring physical touch (by way of holding hands, a hand on your shoulder or stroking your arm) can connect you as a birth team. This can start whilst your spinal anaesthetic is being administered and continue once you're lying down preparing for birth.

I believe that any birth experience can be improved and feel more connected if the woman or birthing person:

- Feels safe.
- Feels listened to.
- Trusts their body's ability to birth and heal.
- Is supported by people supporting their choices.
- Feels confident about making decisions and advocating for themselves.
- Has tools to make them feel calmer and more comfortable – even happy!

And hypnobirthing puts a big tick against all of that and more.

Putting hypnobirthing into practice

At every stage of your journey there are opportunities to use the skills, techniques and mind-body connection knowledge gained through hypnobirthing.

During pregnancy

Something you can start at any time is listening to *hypnobirthing audio tracks*. I have my own album, which I gift to my clients and sell on my website, but you can search online for single tracks or albums to purchase. Listening to hypnobirthing audios (which is a form of self-hypnosis; a state where you're fully in control but able to fully relax) allows you to switch off your conscious brain and begin to reframe any limiting beliefs you may have about birth or yourself. They encourage you to see the bigger picture, release fear and come to realise what you're capable of. The cumulative effect of this regular, daily auditory practice means you'll be building strength, resilience and a sense of calm confidence.

Positive affirmations can be used daily in pregnancy to reprogram your inner thoughts about your pregnancy, birth or postnatal journey. The 'feelings region' in your subconscious mind is great at absorbing messages, and it files them away in case it needs them in the future. By showing it messages that are uplifting, reassuring, comforting, strengthening and of a growth-mindset, you're nourishing your mind and focusing on things you *can* control. You may not consciously believe these statements to be true at first, but slowly you'll experience neuroplasticity in action; the building of new neural pathways that help you change your habits, beliefs and mindset. They really can be so powerful.

Pregnancy is the time to practise *making confident and informed decisions*. Through hypnobirthing you'll be developing this skill by looking at evidence, reflecting on what feels right for you and noticing how things make you feel. This is your birth and postnatal experience and there are many choices you'll need to make, even if it feels like there's not much you can impact with a Caesarean birth.

One of the kindest things you can do for yourself in pregnancy is commit to *focusing on what you can control*, and releasing what you can't. This isn't as easy as it sounds! This skill can be adapted to any part of your life and is one you'll learn to hone during your hypnobirthing practice.

Fill your *Hypno-Bubble* with the things that make you feel good, and practise dialling down the noise on things that don't serve you. This bubble can be utilized in hospital to allow you to come inwards and tune into your mind and body.

The support you have around you after baby is born is something to prioritize. Spend this time *curating* your go-to people and resources to deactivate any stress responses about how you'll manage postnatally.

The night before

Eating a delicious meal (ahead of your nil-by-mouth) is a must – but make it mindful. Get the fancy tablecloth and glasses out and honour your last evening before baby arrives. You could spend a few minutes with your eyes closed using *visualization* to think through all the details of the next day and talking about how you want each stage to go. Practising *calming breathing* as you go to bed will help you settle into sleep.

The Birth Day morning

It will be an early start, but listening to a *positive affirmations track* (or reading some *affirmation cards* you have) will ease you into the day and help your mindset. I love the *nostril breath* to help combat nerves and to feel more balanced. Try to notice and tune into what you need and what you're feeling in your body to help you feel grounded.

On the ward

In most cases, you won't know your scheduled birth time until you arrive at the hospital, so mentally prepare to have a fairly long wait until it's your turn. Go armed with things to do/watch/listen to/distract yourself with, keeping in mind what you already know makes you feel safe, calm, happy and in your parasympathetic nervous system. You could certainly focus on your *breathing* when you need it and be *visualizing* your calm and happy place in your mind.

Getting your spinal anaesthetic

Whilst the doctor administers your spinal block, your birth partner or your midwife can help with *reassuring physical touch* if you'd like them to; this could be holding your hand or stroking your arm. The *calming breath* you've learnt and practised will come in handy here, too. If you know you might find this stage challenging, you could have a *positive affirmation* that helps you through which your birth partner or midwife could repeat out loud, or you could be silently repeating to yourself.

During birth

Some people like to chat and laugh through their birth, and others prefer the quiet, maybe even with eyes closed and surrendering to what's coming next. Your *calming breath, affirmations* and *reassuring physical touch* may be weaved in if it feels right. Telling yourself what you're excited for can help combat feelings of any fearful adrenaline that's being produced.

After birth

Noticing your *mind–body connection* after birth is important, but one that will feel strange at first as you won't have the full feeling back in your body for several hours. Everything you've practised in your pregnancy is so relevant to postpartum as your body heals and you continue to move through new milestones. *Positive affirmations, breathing* and *being mindful about movement* can be daily habits. Your environment and 'nest' will be key to your recovery, so consider what you can see, hear, touch, feel, smell and taste to help you slow down and maximise quietness and rest as much as possible. *Releasing fear* isn't just for pregnancy and birth, it's vital to continue this as your instinct to worry or 'look for threat' may be heightened. It goes without saying that a good support network can help you enjoy your fourth trimester (and not just get through it), so it's now time to put everything you planned into action.

Wishing you all the very best on your hypnobirthing for Caesarean birth journey.

My birth story: Imogen

I have had two C-sections. One emergency and one elected. Quite different experiences, but I used hypnobirthing for both.

With my first, a C-section never even crossed my mind when I found out I was pregnant. I planned for a 'natural birth'. I didn't even consider hypnobirthing either, until my NHS midwife recommended it to me. I found Laura, who was local to me and was able to come to my home. With my job in TV, it was hard to find time to attend group sessions.

Again, I originally planned for a 'natural birth' and did all the exercises for pain relief and control. Laura insisted, though, that I keep a C-section at the back of my mind. It probably wouldn't happen, but to be somewhat prepared mentally.

Going forward in my pregnancy, I repeated my mantras – 'take control of what I can and let go of what I can't' – and played my affirmations at night. I felt very prepared.

Then a routine midwife appointment on my due date turned my birth plan on its head. I had suddenly developed pre-eclampsia. I was in complete shock, as I felt fine and the only symptoms I had were my blood pressure and protein in my urine. My blood pressure was increasing rapidly, so it was decided I would need an induction. Unfortunately this sent my womb into hyper stimulation. I managed the pain with my breath techniques and had no medical pain management (gas and air didn't work!). However, things quickly started taking a turn for the worse and I was rushed into an emergency C-section under general anaesthetic.

Now, a lot of people would feel quite traumatized waking up from such an experience. But I just felt elated to meet my baby. I truly let go of what I couldn't control, but also took control in demanding to know everything that was about to happen to me. I made sure I stayed informed throughout the chaos and I kept calm. I used the BRAIN* acronym. Something I had embedded in my mind.

I really believe my hypnobirthing classes prevented me from feeling traumatized and allowed me to feel the baby bubble of love that other mothers feel. I felt connected to my baby still.

With my second pregnancy, it was discovered at 34 weeks that my placenta wasn't performing efficiently. I had to have an elective C-section at 37 weeks to prevent anything happening to my baby. I was quite negative about what was going to happen and stopped being excited to have a baby. I booked in a recap session with the view that I would most likely be having another C-section, which I didn't want. But after my refresher session, I felt a lot more informed and felt confident enough to ensure it happened on my terms.

This C-section was very positive and I felt in control and calm. And again, I let go of what I wasn't in control of.

I now have two healthy babies with, what feels to me, non-traumatic births. I always recommend to anyone having a baby to try hypnobirthing. You're not just preparing for the pain, you're preparing your mind for what is going to happen, good or bad. Sadly, you can't always have complete control of what your body does, but you can control how your mind reacts to this.

*The acronym BRAIN is a decision-making tool that can help people make informed choices about their pregnancy or care:

- **B:** Benefits: What are the benefits of making this decision?
- **R:** Risks: What are the risks associated with this decision?
- **A:** Alternatives: Are there any alternatives?
- **I:** Intuition: How do I feel? What is my gut feeling about a decision?
- **N:** Nothing: What if I decide to do nothing/wait and see?

4

What to expect from your C-section operation

If you have a C-section delivery it will either be an elective (planned) C-section or an emergency operation. This chapter explains what to expect in either eventuality. For more information on the differences between these types of C-sections please refer to Chapter 1 on different types of C-sections.

What to expect during an elective C-section operation

Pre-operative appointment

During the week before your scheduled C-section you will be asked to attend a pre-operative appointment. This appointment will give you the chance to ask any questions about the procedure, so go prepared with a list of questions. A member of the team will explain what to expect from the procedure and make sure you have any necessary pre-operative medications that are needed. This may include antibiotics, anti-sickness medicine and antacids to reduce the acidity of your stomach. They will also perform some blood tests to check your iron levels, blood type and antibody screen (in case you need a blood transfusion).

They'll let you know whether your operation is in the morning or afternoon, but you may want to find out how many women are scheduled before you to give you an idea of potential delays. Usually only around two to three are planned per day to allow time for emergency C-sections.

You will need to fast before your operation, so they will let you know from which time you need to do this, including when you can drink water until, and when you should arrive at the hospital.

Questions to ask at your pre-operative appointment

We've answered some of these questions later on in this chapter, but some things you may want to ask are:

- Should I shave or trim my pubic hair before coming in for my operation?
- Where am I on the list of scheduled C-sections?
- How many people are expected in theatre?
- Will there be any students in the theatre?
- Can my partner stay with me the whole time?
- Can I bring a playlist?
- How long should I expect to wait before meeting my baby?
- How long should I expect the full operation to take?
- Can I breastfeed in the theatre?
- Can I have skin-to-skin in the theatre?
- Can I have the screen down when my baby is being born?
- Will my partner be able to cut the cord?
- Can I have delayed cord clamping?
- Can I do vaginal seeding?
- What type of wound closure should I expect, and why are they choosing that option?

Going into hospital
Before you leave home

- Make sure you have a shower at home before going into the hospital using a body wash, paying particular attention to your pubic region and abdomen, and don't use any moisturizers or creams on the area after.
- You will be asked to remove all your jewellery, piercings, false nails and potentially makeup so it's best to do this at home to keep your valuables safe.
- Hair removal – speak to your medical team before doing this as shaving in the days before your operation may increase your chances of infection. Find out if they do want you to remove your hair and if so, do it with clippers rather than a razor to avoid small breaks in the skin.

At the hospital

- You will arrive usually at least a couple of hours before your scheduled operation time and be taken to a waiting area or to your bed.
- Both your anaesthetist (who will be providing your anaesthetic to make you numb and look after you during the operation) and your obstetrician (the doctor who will be performing your surgery) will come round to speak to you and complete the necessary pre-delivery checks and get you to read and sign a consent form.
- You will be given a hospital gown and compression socks to change into, and your birth partner will need to change into scrubs.
- When it's time, a theatre nurse will come and collect you both and take you down to theatre.

This period can be a bit nerve-wracking, so having plenty of entertainment and distractions with you is a really great idea.

During the elective C-section

- Being a planned C-section, the theatre room should feel very calm. Before anything begins you should be able to put your playlist on and familiarize yourself with the room.
- The first person you will usually see is your anaesthetist, who will make you feel comfortable and get you ready to insert your spinal block (other anaesthetics are used but this is the most common, especially during a planned C-section). This involves you sitting on the side of the bed, bending forward and hugging a cushion. The anaesthetist will then insert a needle between two of your vertebrae in the lower part of your spine to administer the anaesthetic. This will numb you from your chest down so that you can be awake during the operation, but not feel any pain.
- You will then be helped to lie down on the operating table and your birth partner will be able to sit right next to your head and be able to support and talk to you throughout the birth. This is something you can plan for and discuss with your partner beforehand; how they can best help you on the day.
- All members of the team who are involved in the operation will then enter the room and will introduce themselves to you.
- It will take from five to 20 minutes for the spinal to be fully effective, and in this time a catheter – a thin, flexible tube that you won't be

able to feel – will be inserted into your bladder. The anaesthetic can make you feel shaky but this is normal, and your anaesthetist will check in with you regularly to check how you're feeling.

- You will also have a cannula inserted, usually in the back of your hand or arm so that you can be given fluids and other medicines intravenously (straight into your blood system).
- A screen will be placed in front of you so that you can't see the operation being performed.
- Your skin will be cleaned.
- Pubic hair may be cut or shaved where they intend to make the incision.
- The surgeons will ensure you are fully numb before beginning the operation.
- Most commonly, a horizontal cut will be made along your bikini line, your abdominal muscles will be parted along your midline, then a second cut will be made on your uterus.
- As your surgeon helps your baby to be born you may feel some pressure, pulling and tugging from your chest down to your pubic area, but it's not painful.
- For a straightforward, planned C-section you should expect the operation to take around 45 minutes, but you will be able to meet your baby as soon as 20 minutes into the procedure. This may be longer for subsequent Caesareans as they may need to remove scar tissue before delivering the baby.
- Your partner is usually able to stand at the screen and watch/take photos of the baby being born and may be able to cut the cord too.
- Provided everything has gone well, you will be able to hold your baby immediately for skin-to-skin or in a blanket, or your partner can.
- Your surgeon will then remove the placenta and close your wound.

What to expect during an emergency C-section – how is it different from a planned C-section?

Emergency C-sections can be very similar to planned Caesarean births, but here's how it may be different:

- The chats that are usually held with your obstetrician and anaesthetist prior to your operation are likely to be more rushed.

- You (or possibly your birth partner in Category 1 cases) still need to consent to the procedure. This may need to be done verbally as opposed to you being able to read through and sign your consent.
- Like an elective C-section, in most cases you will be able to have a spinal or epidural anaesthetic, or if you have already had an epidural they can often just top this up, which is as effective. Rarely, if a Category 1 C-section is determined you may need to be put under a general anaesthetic, which means you will be asleep whilst your baby is born and your partner will not be able to be in the room either.
- The blood tests that are usually performed a few days before a planned C-section will be done once your cannula is inserted.
- Under a Category 3 or 2, the operation itself will take a similar time to that of a planned C-section but Category 1s are often performed much quicker, and can be done within 30 mins of the decision being made.
- Usually the incision will be made along the bikini line as it is during a planned C-section, but under some circumstances, your surgeon may decide to do a vertical cut instead as it gives quicker access to the baby.
- Depending on the reason for your emergency C-section, your baby may need to be checked by the neonatal team immediately after birth. If everything is fine the baby may be passed to you or your partner (unless you had a general anaesthetic, in which case this would have to be to your partner) but if there are any complications they may be taken to the special care baby unit.

What happens after a C-section?

- Once your C-section procedure is complete, all being well, you, your baby and your birth partner will be taken to a recovery room.
- You will then either be offered some food and drink or be able to eat something you have brought in.
- You will remain here for around an hour or so whilst the medical staff perform regular checks on you.
- You will be offered pain medication, treatment to reduce the risk of blood clots like your compression socks and injections of medicine (usually into your abdomen).
- Your midwife will also be able to help you with breastfeeding if you have chosen to breastfeed.

Once they are happy that you are stable, you will be moved to the ward where you will remain for the rest of your stay.

On the ward

- Your catheter will remain in place usually for around 12 hours until you are able to stand and move around.
- You will be encouraged to get up and move around and go to the toilet as soon as six hours after your operation.
- Regular pain relief will be continually offered to you throughout your stay.
- Your wound will be covered by a dressing that will stay in place for at least 24 hours but possibly longer, depending on your medical team's advice.
- Your baby will be next to you and you'll be able to have regular close contact and support with feeding.
- If everything has gone well you should expect to be in hospital for one to two days; if there are any complications that require a longer stay you will be advised of this.
- If your baby is taken to the neonatal unit, you will need to wait till you're well enough to be able to go and see them, which can be difficult.

Is it harder to recover from an emergency C-section?

Depending on your circumstances, if you've had an emergency C-section as opposed to a planned one, you may feel a lot more exhausted and depleted. You may find it harder to recover from this due to:

- Having gone through a long labour prior to your C-section. This can be exhausting, and of course you're going to feel more fatigued and weak once your baby is born. The physical and emotional toll of labour adds up, making recovery a bit more challenging.
- Having been in hospital for a few days. If you were induced, or if you or baby needed extra monitoring for health concerns, then you may have already been in hospital for a number of days or weeks. The hospital environment, though necessary for care, isn't always the most restful. The constant activity, lack of fresh air, and the general

stress of being in a medical setting can leave you feeling drained, affecting both your physical and emotional recovery.

- Stress and lack of sleep are other factors that can impact your recovery. If you've been through a challenging and possibly life-threatening birth experience this can be both mentally and emotionally taxing. It's important to remember that this stress can influence how quickly and smoothly you recuperate.
- Previous health issues play a role, too. If you were dealing with medical conditions such as pre-eclampsia, uncontrolled diabetes, or any illness that made you feel unwell before your C-section, your body might need extra time and care to recover. These pre-existing challenges can make the postpartum period more demanding.

Of course, not every experience will be the same, but this is a good guide of what to expect so as to help you to prepare. Part of the reason we recommend being well-informed about Caesarean births, even if it's not your preferred birth option, is because only a small percentage of C-section births in the UK are elective. In a potentially fraught situation, it can feel overwhelming and difficult to make decisions, and in some cases those decisions may fall to your birth partner. Having discussions about your preferences should a C-section be necessary, with your partner ahead of time, means it is more likely that you will be more comfortable with your birth experience. Regarding long-term physical and emotional recovery, the outcomes are usually better for people who felt they maintained control and were able to still implement some of their own preferences throughout their birth.

My birth story: Amber

I fell pregnant in November 2022 and was hoping for a healthy and uncomplicated pregnancy, but due to having ulcerative colitis (inflammatory bowel disease) I was told I'd need to be under consultant care with regular scans and appointments throughout the second half of my pregnancy. Due to my UC and previous complications, I knew a C-section would be the best option for me.

I had my first consultant appointment in which I explained my concerns for a vaginal birth and my preference for a C-section.

After a bit of back and forth (they felt a vaginal birth was still safe for me but ultimately, I knew my own body), they agreed to go ahead with this option.

My C-section was booked for Monday 24 July, so I attended the hospital the Friday prior for the pre-op. I'll be honest, at this point I was majorly nervous. They have to go into a lot of detail around what's involved as well as the risks to you/baby, so it feels a lot! It didn't help that my husband was starting to feel dizzy in the corner listening to all the info ...

The morning of the C-section I arrived at 7.30 a.m. I was taken to the elective C-section ward where a bed was ready as well as the cot for the baby (very surreal!). We had numerous midwives come and introduce themselves to us, as well as the surgeon who would be performing the C-section. This all felt very organized and reassuring.

I was first on the list, so by 8.15 I was making my way down to theatre. When I entered the room, the nerves really came over me. Everyone was so incredibly supportive and reassuring, and I really did feel like I was in the best hands. We had made a Spotify playlist, which they connected to a speaker in the theatre – we were then all just chatting about song choices and the cheesy music we'd picked – it was so calm and positive, which put me at ease instantly.

I then sat down on the bed and the anaesthetist talked me through everything, put my cannula in and then carried out the spinal block. My husband was sitting in front of me holding my hand the whole time and I had a midwife there supporting me.

Once the spinal block was complete, I laid down and my catheter was fitted; I couldn't feel this at all as the numbness had already kicked in. The surgeon told me that they would start, and within a few minutes our baby would be born. They pinned my gown up in front so we couldn't see anything, and my husband sat by my head and held my hand as we anxiously waited to meet our baby boy.

Five or ten minutes later we heard a cry, and our baby was here; they peered him over the gown and then asked if I wanted to hold him straightaway or if I was happy for them to clean him up and bring him to me – I opted for the latter, as I really did feel quite exhausted by this point, so my husband held him. The midwives took lots of pictures for us and then brought my baby over to me to have skin-to-skin – during this time the surgeons were stitching me. This was probably the hardest part of the procedure as it did feel like it took a long time, but I was holding my baby, which was a good distraction. I was in theatre for about an hour and then wheeled back onto the ward where I was offered tea and toast.

After a few hours the spinal started to wear off, and I regained feeling in my legs, my catheter was removed, and I was able to go to the toilet. Standing up for the first time felt very strange, and it was a very slow shuffle to the bathroom and back – my tip for that first walk out of bed is to take pain relief about 30 minutes before, to make it more bearable.

I was discharged the following day and, when we got home, I spent as much time as I could in bed having skin-to-skin and breastfeeding, and my husband did all the nappies (winning!) and took care of us both. The first two to three days were the hardest in terms of mobility and pain, but if I stayed on top of pain relief it was manageable. I could hold my baby comfortably from the start and after five days I took my first walk outdoors – it was about ten minutes and very steady, but it felt good to have some fresh air. By week three, I was comfortably walking 20–30 minutes at a time.

After about 6–8 weeks I started scar massage regularly, which improved numbness instantly. I did this daily for a couple of months and then a few times a week. My baby is now 13 months old, and I think my scar has healed very well and I have very little numbness in the area.

My C-section experience and recovery has been very positive, and I plan to have another elective C-section if we ever have a second baby.

5

Different types of anaesthetics for your C-section operation

When you go in for a C-section, the first step once you're in the operating room is having your anaesthetic, which is a type of medicine that ensures you won't feel any pain during the surgery. The most common types used are spinal or epidural anaesthetics. These work by numbing your body from the chest down. Despite this numbness, you'll remain awake and fully aware of what's happening around you. This means that, although you won't feel any pain, you'll be able to experience your baby's birth and, all being well, be able to hold them immediately.

Most C-sections are performed in this way because it's generally safer for both the mother and the baby. Additionally, it enables your birth partner to accompany you, allowing you to experience the birth of your child together.

What's the difference between a spinal and an epidural anaesthetic?

An epidural is most often used to provide pain relief during labour without affecting your ability to move your legs or push your baby out. Your spinal cord and nerves are contained in a sac of cerebrospinal fluid and the (potential) space around this sac is called the epidural space which also contains veins, fat and nerve roots. It's here in the epidural space that the anaesthetic injection is placed via a thin plastic tube. This helps in controlling the effects of the medicine and the speed at which it works, which is ideal when being used as pain relief only, and so you don't lose the feeling in your legs.

An epidural is a catheter, essentially like a little tap that enables the medicine to be topped up if needed. An epidural would usually only be used as anaesthetic for your C-section if you had already had one inserted during labour, which eventually results in a C-section, as the epidural would simply be topped up. It does however take longer to be effective because of its placement, and will usually require a larger amount of anaesthetic than would be used for a spinal.

A spinal anaesthetic refers to when the anaesthetic is given directly into the sac where your spinal cord and nerves are contained. A spinal block would usually be used in an elective C-section or if you hadn't already had an epidural in your earlier labour. It can also be given if you've had an epidural that isn't working well enough to give good enough anaesthesia for a C-section. For the block to be given, you will be asked to sit on the side of the bed with your feet on a stool. You will then need to bend forward over a pillow and create a curve in your back so that your anaesthetist has some space between the bones of your spine to insert the needle. First a very fine needle is used to inject a mixture of local anaesthetic and pain relief so that you won't feel the spinal block happening, shortly followed by the spinal injection itself.

Spinals and epidurals do have the same effect in numbing the lower part of your body, but because the spinal is more direct, the effect of it is immediate.

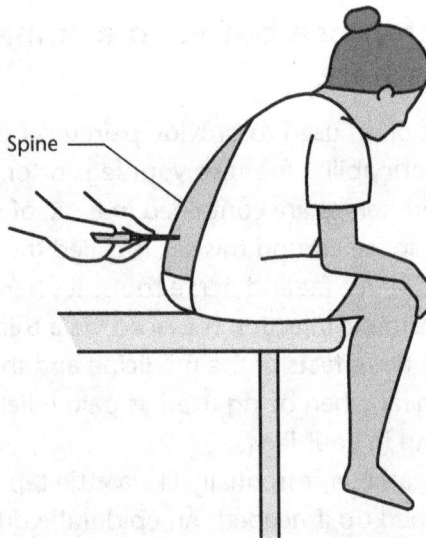

Figure 5.1 A spinal block is administered in preparation for a C-section

Sometimes a combined spinal-epidural is used where you have the advantages of the quick effects of a spinal injection and the advantage of an epidural catheter, so that the medicine can be topped up easily if needed.

Will I know if my anaesthetic is working or not?

Once the anaesthesia is administered, your anaesthetist will help you to lie down on the operating bed. You will quickly start to feel a warming or tingling sensation starting in your feet and moving up through your body to your chest. This is followed by your feet and legs becoming numb and heavy to the point where you can't move them. It's typical to experience numbness from your lower chest down, but this won't impact your ability to breathe, although you might feel a bit short of breath. Feeling shaky is also normal. You can be assured that the quality of the numbing block will be checked by the anaesthetist before they let the surgery start to make sure it is working well enough, which they check with a cold spray or a cold stick. Your cold and pain nerves run together, so if you can't feel the cold, you won't be able to feel the incision. Throughout the surgery, your anaesthetist will be right beside you. You can speak to them and ask any questions, and they'll be closely monitoring your vital signs like blood pressure, oxygen levels and heart rate, as well as making sure you are comfortable and pain-free throughout.

General anaesthetic

This is when you are asleep (unconscious) whilst the Caesarean operation is performed. This type of anaesthetic is only used if this is the safest choice for you and baby for specific medical or other reasons. This includes: having an abnormal spine, which may mean the spinal block can't be administered; if you have a condition where your blood cannot clot properly; or if the spinal or epidural doesn't work properly. It may also be used if an urgent C-section is required to deliver your baby as quickly as possible. Even with emergency C-section operations, a general anaesthetic is still mostly only usually used in a Category 1 emergency situation (explained in more detail in Chapter 1 on types of C-sections).

Occasionally spinal blocks also fail to provide enough anaesthetic to keep you pain-free during the operation (remember, your anaesthetist will always check this before any surgery begins), in which instance a general anaesthetic would also be used. If you have a general anaesthetic you will be asleep during the birth of your baby, and your birth partner will also have to wait outside while you're in the operating theatre. But, all being well with the baby, they will be able to hold them almost immediately whilst you come round from surgery.

Mothers often worry that the anaesthetic may have a negative impact on their baby, but actually the medicine given to induce sleep during surgery is known to have little effect on the baby. It's rare for the amount of anaesthetic required to reach the baby's brain, and the procedure is considered safe for infants.

To ease your concerns, it's a good idea to have conversations with your midwife or OBGYN and birthing team prior to your delivery date, so that you can ask any questions or seek reassurance about any part of the procedure in advance. This is likely to really help you to feel more calm on the day and enjoy the remainder of your pregnancy. In the case of an emergency C-section, you may not have had much time to ask so many questions, but similarly, preparing for a possibility of a C-section birth, even if it is not your ideal plan, can significantly influence how the situation plays out on the day.

More information on epidurals can be found here: https://www.labourpains.org/.

6

Types of C-section incisions and closures

The most common type of C-section cut is performed horizontally, around 2–3 cm above your pubic bone and is approximately 15–20 cm long. You will find that the exact location of this will vary between women, with some cuts lower than others. This is often down to the surgeon's preference and may be impacted by the woman's body shape and size, with some plus-size women having cuts higher up to potentially limit overhang and improve healing. It could also be influenced by the position of the placenta and the position of the baby, and whether you have had previous abdominal surgeries too.

Rarely, a vertical cut is made instead, as it provides faster access to the baby in emergency situations or due to previous abdominal surgeries.

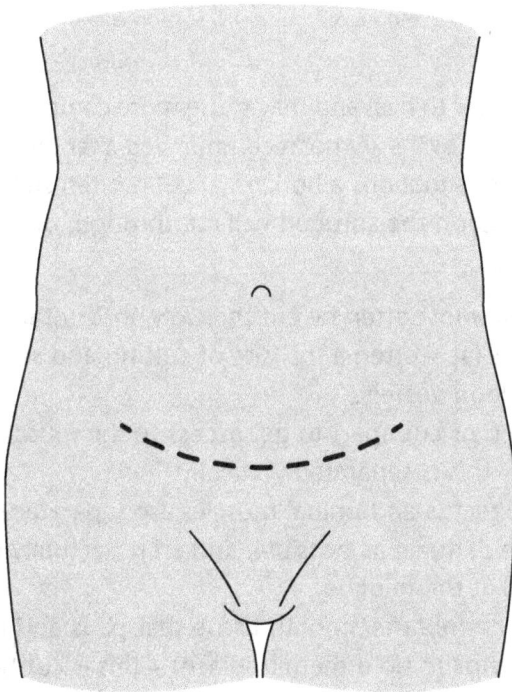

Figure 6.1 Horizontal C-section cut

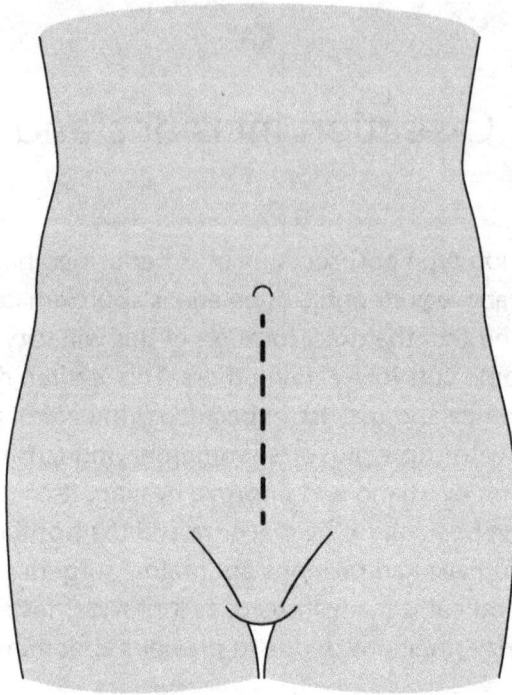

Figure 6.2 Vertical C-section cut

But, as it takes longer to heal and may cause more complications in future pregnancies (vaginal births are not recommended after this type of incision), even in emergency situations a horizontal cut is often still used.

During a C-section the surgeon will cut through, or separate, seven layers of tissue:

- Skin – this will most often be cut through horizontally.
- Subcutaneous fat – often a mixture of cutting and separating to limit damage to blood vessels.
- Fascia – pulled or cut apart to get access to the muscle layer underneath – this is separated vertically.
- Muscle – the rectus abdominal muscles are separated vertically to cause as little damage as possible, and aren't actually cut through but stretched at the midline.
- Peritoneum (membrane/smooth tissue that pads and insulates your organs and helps to hold them in place) – this is cut horizontally and pushed down to expose the uterus.

- Uterus – this is cut and separated to reveal the amniotic sac.
- Amniotic sac – carefully cut open to birth your baby.

When closing you back up again, the surgeon will stitch in a way to prevent a hernia, and for the best healing outcome for you. The uterus is usually closed with two layers of dissolvable stitches to provide additional support for any future pregnancies. The surgeon may or may not stitch together your muscles and fat layer, as it can have a better outcome when these layers are left to heal by themselves. Your skin surface will then be closed with one of the methods below.

Types of skin closures

Each surgeon will have their own preference for skin closure, and this may differ by location and the health of the mother.

There are two main types of skin closure following a C-section:

Surgical stitches – which can be done with either absorbable or non-dissolvable thread; this can take an extra 30 minutes compared to using staples.

Surgical staples – these are the quickest method of wound closure and typically would be used when quick closure is required, i.e. if the mother is unwell and they need to close the wound quickly to focus their attention elsewhere.

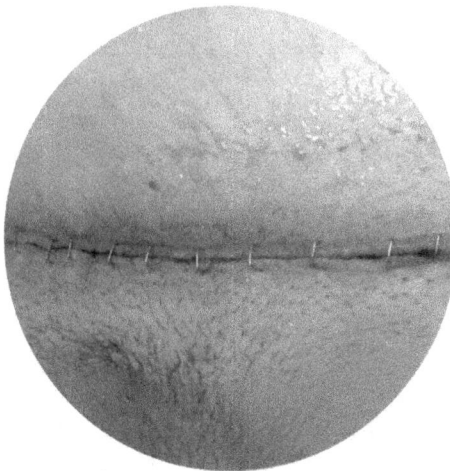

Figure 6.3 Surgical staples after a C-section operation

Helpers

Surgical glue – is usually applied over the top of stitches to seal the wound and help prevent infections. It will gradually peel off as the wound heels

Steri strips – can be placed over the top of the stitches as well to provide additional support.

A dressing will then be placed over your wound. Again, the surgeon will have their own preference as to the type of dressing they use.

If you have a preference over what type of skin closure and dressing is used, you can absolutely speak to your doctor at your pre-operative appointment (if you're having an elective C-section). But it's also OK to ask even if you're having an emergency C-section.

7

Early C-section scar care

Early scar care can make a big difference to the outcome of your scar and your recovery. You're more likely to have a non-problematic scar, as well as a more aesthetically pleasing scar – a flatter, less red scar with less chance of an overhang – if you prioritize early scar healing.

The longer a wound takes to heal, the more scar tissue is likely to form, so knowing how to rest, recover and care for your wound well is so important.

The acute healing phase (the time it takes for your wound to heal and close over) will last approximately 6–8 weeks, but it's completely normal to still feel pain, numbness and sensitivity for longer. It takes six months for a scar to fully 'heal' and form, and up to two years for it to completely mature (possibly even longer). So you can see why it may still be causing issues months or years later, particularly if left untreated or if you've neglected good wound care at the start.

Scar care information is the same for all scars, regardless of whether they are horizontal or vertical. It may just take a bit longer if your scar isn't in the classical horizontal position, and you may need to air a horizontal scar more, particularly if you have an overhang.

Mobilizing the scar tissue whilst it's healing helps the scar tissue lay down in a more uniform pattern, meaning you are likely to have less scar tissue, and a scar that moves more freely and looks better. A better-moving scar, with fewer restrictions or adhesions and less tension, also means the scar will have less of an impact on the rest of your body too.

Fascia is a layer of connective tissue that covers the whole body, keeping muscles, organs, nerves, bones and blood vessels in place. It plays a role in supporting good circulation, reduces friction between layers of soft tissue and has its own nerve supply, so can become irritated or hypersensitive. Often, scars can put tension on the fascia of the body because the scar interrupts the normal gliding movement of the fascia over other tissues. A C-section scar at the abdominal or pelvic region can cause the body to be pulled forward and down towards the scar, shortening through the front of the body and causing tension, which can lead to issues such as back, hip and shoulder pain.

Touching your scar as soon as possible (with clean hands and or through clothes) will also help to stimulate the nerves in the area that have been damaged and help to prevent numbness or hypersensitivity and restore any loss of sensation as soon as possible. We recommend you to try to interact with your scar as soon as you can, even if this just means looking at it at first. So many women report not ever interacting with their scars, even years after their birth. This may be due to it triggering negative feelings about their birth, or feeling squeamish about the wound, but often a lack of engagement with your scar does lead to other problems as you recover. For example, the muscles and nerves in the area also switching off, or functioning poorly, leaving you at a greater risk of injury, ongoing numbness and sensitivity or a pooch appearance. If you are struggling with negative feelings about your birth, which affects your ability to engage with your scar, please turn to Chapter 18 on birth trauma.

In Chapter 9, on what to expect after a C-section, you can read all about how you are likely to feel after your C-section and how best you can recover.

Signs of infection

Particularly in the early days, it's really important to know and watch for the signs of an infection. The sooner you can get treatment the fewer issues this will cause generally, and you'll have a better outcome in terms of the amount of scar tissue you end up with, pain and how the scar looks. Contact your midwife or a GP straight away if you have any of the following symptoms after a Caesarean:

- Heat
- Redness
- Odour
- Oozing from the site – clear or yellow/green discharge
- Generally feeling unwell in yourself
- A temperature.

Wound closure

Most commonly, dissolvable stitches are used to close the wound but occasionally non-absorbing stitches or staples are used and you will need to go and get these removed. You should be given this information before leaving hospital, if you're unsure, just ask before you're discharged.

If you have dissolvable stitches and/or glue, there's no need to rub at them, they will come off in time in the shower, or by gently applying scar oil.

If you've had staples you will find you have small dots left either side of your scar but these should fade in time especially with scar massage, a good scar oil and silicone.

Caring for your wound/scar

With most dressings, it's fine to take a shower, but don't submerge the area in a bath. Often your dressing will be clear so you can easily keep an eye out for any bleeding or oozing from the wound. It's a good idea to look at it regularly so you can watch for changes.

Once your dressing has been removed, it's really important to keep the area clean and dry. The best way to do this is:

- Wear loose, breathable clothing to allow air to circulate to the wound or nothing at all for periods of the day if you can.
- Stick to showering over bathing.
- To wash with clean water only from the shower. Things like washes and surgical spirits can cause irritation and you're more likely to get an infection.
- Avoid pool or sea swimming until your wound is fully closed over.
- To pat the wound dry with a fresh, clean towel after showering.
- If you have an overhang, you may want to use some sterile gauze in the fold to soak up any excess moisture.
- With plus-sized tummy, you may also benefit from some time laid down to get air to the area.

We have some top tips below for plus-sized tummies and an overhang.

You need to keep the wound area clean, and the best way to do this is to wash the scar area daily with the shower head on a gentle setting, lifting your tummy to wash underneath if needed. You don't need to use any products on it to clean it, water alone is enough. It's advisable not to bathe or swim until your wound is closed over, if the area is very sensitive or irritable or if you struggle to dry it properly. When you do return to bathing, make sure the bath is clean before filling it. It's the same with showering: avoid using any bath products such as bubble baths until your wound is fully closed and scab free.

Top tips for recovery with a C-section overhang

Having a tummy that folds over your wound site can increase the risk of an infection and complications after having a C-section. But there are a number of things you can do to help your scar heal well if you have an overhang.

- If it's possible, you may want to discuss with your surgeon prior to surgery what they suggest in terms of where the incision is made, which skin-closure type is used and any post-op things that can be done to improve your healing.
- Pico dressings are great for aiding healing. These dressings use negative pressure to draw out excess fluid from the wound whilst also protecting the incision. The absorbent dressing is attached to a pump which, when turned on, pulls the air out of the dressing and the excess fluid from the wound is pulled into the dressing. The dressing helps to prevent bacteria from entering the wound and the negative pressure can improve blood flow, helping the wound to heal. Usually if your doctor thinks this type of dressing is necessary for you it will be applied. But if you have a larger tummy, you may want to ask your surgeon about this prior to surgery to find out if they are planning on using one, and you can absolutely request it too.
- With an overhang, it can be hard to keep the area dry. It's especially important that, after your daily shower, you thoroughly dry the wound area either with a clean dry towel or by lying down and lifting your tummy to fully allow the area to air dry before getting dressed. Moist areas are prone to bacteria.

- It's common with an overhang to get sweaty in the fold so if you find the areas getting hot and sweaty, you can use place some sterile gauze in the skin fold to keep the area dry.
- Once the wound is fully healed you can use cornflour as a talc alternative to keep the area dry.
- Medihoney barrier cream is a great option for treating odours from the area, preventing chafing, fungal infections and skin irritation. This product is only suitable on wounds that are closed, so use the Medihoney HCS patches or Medihoney wound gel prior to this to speed up recovery.

As always, if you are struggling with a slow-healing wound or issues with your scar because of your overhang, please seek medical help from your doctor and request to be referred to a wound care specialist if necessary.

Movement

Whilst some movement is useful to promote good healing and to create a scar that moves well with the rest of your body and doesn't cause any tightness or restrictions, your focus should be on rest to allow your body to do what it needs to do to heal well. To find out what movement is beneficial in this early stage see Chapter 21 on early movement to heal and mobilize a scar.

Breathwork can be a lovely tool to gently introduce some movement for your scar without putting any strain on the area. Through your clothes, place your hands gently over your scar and breathe into them, allowing your ribs and tummy to expand. As you take a deep breath in through your nose, your scar and hands should gently rise and fall as you breathe, which helps to get the scar moving as well as encouraging more blood flow to the area and encourage draining of fluid and swelling after surgery.

Video: Diaphragmatic Breathing Tutorial #1

Please use the QR code to visit our physio-led exercise library.

www.youtube.com/@the360mama/videos

Massage

Massaging over the actual scar site is not appropriate until it is healed (scab free and fully closed), but light massage around the abdomen away from and towards the scar can help to promote and speed up healing. Please see Chapter 24 on scar massage for more information on how to do this.

Hydration and nutrition

These play such an important part in early scar recovery and healing. Hydrating well will help the body flush out all the waste product and medications used during your operation. Good nutrition helps to bring the body out of the inflammation process and provide it with the energy and nutrients it needs to heal well. Please head to Chapter 8 to find out more, and for what to eat to optimize recovery.

Slow-healing wounds

You should expect your wound to be closed over by 6–8 weeks post-birth. If this isn't the case, the first thing we'd recommend is to go back to your doctor and get them to check the wound to see if anything is preventing it from closing (like an infection), and they should be able to advise you on how best to help it heal. Remember, you can always request to be referred to see a wound care specialist nurse, which may be a better option. If you head to Chapter 11 on C-section recovery products, you will see that Medihoney is a great product that is widely used in hospitals to speed up healing and help close a slow-healing wound.

Hydration/scar oils and creams

Not only do you need to hydrate your body well by drinking plenty of fluids, but your wound area needs additional hydration too. Wounds lose a lot more moisture than 'normal' tissue, and need additional hydration to heal well. Poor hydration is one of the main causes of abnormal scar healing. Whilst you don't want a damp or moist scar area from contact with water, which can breed bacteria and increase your risk of a fungal infection, using an oil that is safe to use and creates the correct environment for good healing, can speed up recovery and give you a much better outcome with your scar. As well as the Medihoney that can be used from day one post-birth, there are oils that can be used from week two (14 days after birth) to aid healing and get that essential hydration to the scar. Please see Chapter 11 on C-section recovery products for information about which ones are appropriate.

Once you get to six weeks post-birth and your scar is fully closed, it's safe to use most oils on the area (and recommended to do so). However, perfumed oils can irritate your scar and dry out the area causing a tighter scar, so it is best to avoid them.

Studies have shown that using an oil two to three times a day, particularly in the early stages of healing, in the first six months post-op, improves the look, colour and also the quality of the scar tissue (it's still effective and beneficial after this time too.) Oils with ingredients that have been proven to improve scars are best – please see Chapter 11 on C-section recovery products for our favourites.

To apply your oil or cream, make sure the scar area is clean and dry; you just need a small amount of the product, and can gently smear it along the length of your scar with a clean, dry finger. These products are also great on stretch marks too.

Itching after a C-section

This is really common after a surgery and is due to a number of factors:

- The nerves in the area are trying to regenerate and heal, which our body perceives as itching.
- Dryness – if the scar area is dry it can be itchy.
- Histamine is released in the body in response to the injury, which the nerves respond to; again this creates an itchy sensation.

Avoid scratching the area as this will only irritate it further and potentially cause skin damage and infection.

How to treat it

Usually the itching will stop when the remodelling phase of the scar site occurs, around four weeks after birth, however the following can help treat itching:

- A good scar cream/oil will hydrate the area, treating any dryness that's causing the itching but also providing a cooling, soothing effect to the area.
- Silicone strips – like the creams/oils, they hydrate the area and the light compression can be soothing on the scar area. These can be used from six weeks. Before this you can use silicone dressings.
- An ice pack placed over the area can help cool and soothe.
- Compression underwear such as the silicone strips applies light pressure to the area, which can alleviate itching.
- Massage – some people find the itching can go on for months or even years post-birth. if your scar area continues to itch, massage can help to calm the nerve endings and stop the itching – see Chapter 24 on scar massage.
- If the scar area is slow to heal, focusing on everything we've said above to improve healing and get the scar out of the acute healing phase will improve the itching.

Numbness/hypersensitivity

Just like the itching, it's common to experience numbness at the scar site and around it, or even hypersensitivity, when even clothes brushing against the area is too much. This is because nerves have been disrupted or severed in the area: either they need some stimulation to restore feeling, or they need calming to settle. Both numbness and hypersensitivity can often be treated through massage, movement and breathwork. We cover this in more depth in Chapter 24 on scar massage, but in the early days, the best thing you can do is some breathwork with your hands over your scar, and some really light touches of the area above and towards the scar. This encourages those nerve endings to regenerate as soon as possible, and prevent these issues from becoming an ongoing problem.

UV protection

Scar tissue is much more prone to sun damage than regular skin and needs to be protected from UV radiation, especially in the first 12 to 24 months. Scars that are exposed to UV rays are likely to become darker, thicker, more obvious and are more likely to burn. Make sure your scar is always covered with an appropriate fabric (the silicone strips we recommend also provide excellent UV protection) and once healed, still try to avoid direct sun on the scar area and apply a factor 50 suncream if you're outside.

Why might my scar be taking longer to heal?

The ideal situation is to go into surgery knowing it's going to happen having rested well, eaten and hydrated well so your body is in the best possible position to recover. However, we know that the majority of C-sections are unplanned, and this means most people go into them unprepared, having possibly spent a long time in labour already, leaving them feeling exhausted and depleted. This doesn't mean your recovery will necessarily be harder or longer than someone who's had a planned C-section, it's just to highlight how essential it is to prioritize early recovery and scar care for a good outcome.

There are a number of things that can also increase the risk of wound infection and poor or slow healing:

- Being overweight
- Smoking
- Diabetes
- Poor diet without enough nutrients.

It may not be possible to change these factors immediately, especially if your operation was not planned. However, by following our early scar care and C-section recovery advice, you can reduce the risk of infection occurring, improve your healing and ensure that any issues are spotted quickly.

When to seek help after a C-section

Contact your midwife or a GP straight away if you have any of the following symptoms after a Caesarean:

- Severe pain
- Leaking urine
- Pain when peeing
- Heavy vaginal bleeding
- Vaginal blood or discharge that smells unpleasant
- Your wound becomes redder, painful and swollen
- Discharge of pus or foul-smelling fluid from your wound
- High temperature
- Feeling faint, dizzy or with a fast-pounding heartbeat
- Cough, shortness of breath or chest pain
- Severe headache
- Swelling or pain in your lower leg.

These symptoms may be the sign of an infection or blood clot, which should be treated as soon as possible.

Why scar care matters

Scar care generally is an area of after-care that many people tell us they struggle to find information about after being discharged from hospital. For this reason, so many women will believe that numbness and sensitivity around their scar is 'normal' and will live with the symptoms for years. Caring for your wound and scar properly can be the difference between a scar that looks, feels and functions well in the years afterwards, or one that continues to present problems. If you're reading this ahead of your birth, make a plan that ensures you are prioritizing all the things we've mentioned above, but even if you're reading it later on, be assured that it's never too late to begin treating your scar and still see good results. Keep reading for more detailed instructions about how to make your scar look and feel its best.

My birth story: Romy

This was my first baby. We had been told at our 20-week scan that our baby would be born with an upper limb difference, (it's totally random with no known cause). Otherwise it was a textbook pregnancy, and so I chose to book a home birth. I lost my waters gradually over about a period of a week and eventually ended up in the hospital at 41+4 with mild contractions but no progression of labour. I was offered a hormone drip to help to progress labour but I declined because I was aware of the high likelihood of inter-ventions and emergency C-section rates associated with a birth initiated in this way. And also because it would have to be admin-istered with an epidural, which would mean I was unable to move around the room and I wasn't keen on this. I opted for a C-section instead on my terms.

As soon as I was told we would meet our baby within half an hour of making that decision I felt overwhelmingly excited. I hadn't really absorbed any information during my pregnancy about C-sections as I'd hoped not to have one. Despite this I felt very calm and supported by my partner, particularly as we had done a hypnobirthing course – he was fantastic. Our baby was born to a playlist we had made and breastfed very shortly after being born. We went home the next day with no complications. I didn't feel panicked or stressed at any stage.

The recovery advice in hospital was minimal, but I found good information from friends who had also had C-sections. I focused on keeping the wound clean and using silicone patches. A year later my scar is flat and very pale. I have no functional issues, it has a very slight puff on one end, but it has never been painful or pulling. I made a conscious choice to touch it from the beginning so sensitivity has never been an issue. I would rather not have it but I don't have any negative feelings about it!

It's not at all the birth I thought I'd have, but knowing my options and having an informed partner really helped me feel I had chosen my birth and set me up for a great start to parenting life.

8

Nutrition to support your C-section recovery

How you feed and fuel your body before and after a C-section birth can make a big difference to how your body feels and how quickly you heal. The nutrients you get from your diet will provide your body with the energy required to heal, and the process of building new tissue, regaining strength or recovering from potential blood loss requires specific nutrients best gained through your diet. We know that it can be tempting to rely on fast food or snacks when you are tired and overwhelmed after birth, but eating well really can make a big impact on your overall recovery. We hope to guide you in this chapter to understand better how to plan your diet before and after birth to support your well-being and recovery.

This chapter is kindly contributed by Dr Jenna Macciochi, a Senior Lecturer in Immunology at The University of Sussex and a fitness instructor and health coach. Jenna specializes in the intersection of nutrition, movement, mind-body practices and lifestyle with the immune system in health and disease.

The building blocks of recovery

Nutrition plays a crucial role in the recovery process following a C-section. Proper nutrition can speed up healing, reduce inflammation, and help restore energy levels. The right nutrients support tissue repair, immune function, and overall recovery. Imagine your body as a construction site; after the surgery, it's bustling with activity to repair and rebuild. Good nutrition provides the high-quality materials needed for this important work. Just like a well-organized construction site relies on quality materials and skilled workers, your body depends on nutrient-rich foods to rebuild and regain strength.

In the weeks leading up to your C-section, focusing on a healthy diet packed with nutrient-dense foods is essential, even though it might be challenging during the final stages of pregnancy. Lean proteins like chicken, fish, eggs and legumes are crucial as they help repair tissues and build new cells. Make sure to incorporate plenty of colourful fruits and vegetables, which are rich in essential vitamins and minerals like vitamin C and magnesium – key players in immune support and energy production. Additionally, these vibrant foods are packed with phytonutrients, which are plant-based nutrients that provide anti-inflammatory and antioxidant benefits while nourishing your gut biome. Staying well-hydrated by drinking plenty of water and other hydrating fluids is also important, as it supports all bodily functions and prepares you for the demands of surgery and recovery.

Adding some healthy fats, such as those from avocados, nuts and olive oil, can also help improve nutrient absorption. Foods rich in Omega-3 fatty acids, like salmon and chia seeds, are essential to support brain health for both you and the baby, and provide the raw materials for reducing inflammation which will be key to your recovery.

While a balanced diet is your best source of nutrients, certain supplements can provide an added boost. Prenatal vitamin and mineral supplements specifically designed for pregnancy are important for overall nutrient support. If you don't eat oily fish, Omega-3 supplements from either marine or algae sources can be an alternative. If you're concerned about gut health, especially if you'll be taking antibiotics, choosing a probiotic designed to be taken during and after antibiotics could be a prudent addition to your hospital bag. If your iron levels are low, an iron supplement might be recommended by your healthcare provider to prevent anaemia and support your body's preparation for birth and recovery from surgery. This is particularly important after a C-section, as blood loss during the procedure can significantly reduce iron levels, leading to fatigue and impaired healing. Additionally, incorporating iron-rich foods into your diet can help improve your iron levels. Some iron-rich foods include red meat and legumes like lentils, chickpeas and beans. Always aim to have plant-based iron-rich food with a source of vitamin C to improve absorption e.g., hummus and peppers.

Both prenatally and post-C-section, collagen supplements can be beneficial. Collagen is a protein that plays a vital role in maintaining the structure and integrity of skin, all your connective tissues, muscles and bones. Taking collagen supplements before your C-section can help support your body's tissue repair mechanisms, making it easier for your body to heal post-surgery. After your C-section, continuing with collagen supplements can aid in faster wound healing and reduce the appearance of scars as well as support for your postpartum needs.

A well-stocked freezer can be a lifesaver during those first few weeks at home, especially on the days that feel overwhelming. As a new mum, you'll likely be navigating the challenges of caring for your newborn while feeling tired and perhaps experiencing some pain. In such times, taking care of yourself might not be at the top of your list. However, having nutritious, ready-to-eat meals on hand can make a huge difference. It ensures you get the nourishment you need without the stress of cooking, allowing you to focus on recovery and bonding with your baby.

Consider preparing nutrient-rich meals in advance, like hearty soups, curries or stews loaded with nutritious vegetables. Ensure to add protein-rich foods like chicken, fish, tofu, or legumes to provide essential building blocks for tissue repair. Use bone broth, known for its collagen content and healing properties, as a base for soups and stews. Add grains like quinoa or lentils and beans for their gut-supporting fibre. Fibre is incredibly important after a C-section, primarily because it helps ease bowel movements and prevents constipation. Post-surgery, many women experience difficulties with bowel movements due to the effects of anaesthesia, pain medications, and reduced physical activity. Constipation can lead to straining on the toilet, which is particularly uncomfortable and potentially harmful when recovering from abdominal surgery. Bowel movements post-surgery also help your body clear the effects of medications, so it's very critical to support healing. Incorporating probiotic-rich foods like yoghurt, kefir, sauerkraut, and kimchi are also beneficial for gut health.

After your C-section, you might find your appetite is not quite back to normal. This can be a result of hormones, anaesthesia and disrupted sleep. Having gentle, easy-to-eat snacks can help. Smoothie packs are another quick and nutritious option; simply blend spinach, berries, banana, Greek yoghurt and protein powder for a delicious smoothie. Nuts and seeds offer a convenient snack packed with protein and healthy fats. Pre-made salads with a variety of colourful vegetables and a source of protein can also be a lifesaver when you need something healthy and satisfying in a hurry. Whole grain crackers and hummus or yoghurt, berries and nuts are easy on the stomach and support gut health. Staying hydrated with electrolyte drinks is also crucial to help your body recover and maintain energy levels. Herbal teas, such as chamomile or peppermint, can help you relax and unwind. Peppermint tea, in particular, is known for its ability to relieve bloating and gas, making it a soothing choice after a C-section. Ginger tea is great for soothing nausea.

Food can also be a great comfort during the postpartum period. Warm, creamy porridge with berries and nuts can provide a soothing and nutritious start to your day. Good quality dark chocolate is rich in flavonoids and can be a delightful treat that boosts your mood, and when we feel good, science shows we heal better. However, it's important to be mindful of the types of comfort foods you choose. While it might be tempting to reach for sugary snacks or junk food for instant gratification, these options can have negative impacts on your healing process. Consuming high amounts of sugar and processed foods can lead to inflammation and weaken your immune system, making it harder for your body to recover from surgery. Instead, opt for nutrient-dense foods that provide lasting energy and promote healing.

After birth, a good post-natal multivitamin can help ensure you're getting all the necessary nutrients for recovery. Omega-3 fatty acids are also key to help reduce inflammation and promote healing. Probiotics are especially useful if you've been on antibiotics, as they help restore gut health. Collagen supplements continue to be beneficial post-birth, aiding in skin and tissue repair and supporting overall recovery.

If your healing process is slower than expected, certain foods can provide extra support. Bone broth, rich in collagen, is excellent for tissue repair. Incorporating more vitamin C-rich foods, like berries, citrus fruits and bell peppers, can support immune function and collagen production. Zinc-rich foods, such as meat, shellfish and legumes, also play a crucial role in wound healing.

By focusing on nutrient-rich foods and staying hydrated, you can support your body's healing process and recovery after a C-section. Good hydration facilitates the transportation of nutrients and oxygen to cells for healing, and helps remove waste products speeding up recovery. Remember, every bite counts towards nourishing your body and aiding your recovery.

Recipe suggestions from The 360 Mama

Berry smoothie

1 handful frozen mixed berries

1 banana

1 scoop Greek yoghurt

1 handful spinach leaves

100 ml milk of your choice or coconut water

1 scoop protein powder of your choice

You could choose to add a collagen powder of your choice too.

Add all the ingredients to a blender and blend until smooth.

Overnight oats

1 handful rolled oats

1 banana (mashed)

1 tbsp chia seed

1 tbsp flaxseed

1 tbsp honey or raw maple syrup

1 cup milk of your choice

Mix everything well and place in a container in the fridge overnight. The oats are ready to eat the next morning, and you can add fresh toppings of your choosing, such as:

Dried fruit

Fresh berries

Coconut flakes

Nut butter

Seeds

Grated dark chocolate

Lentil soup

1 medium diced onion

1 cup dried red or brown lentils

1 large diced carrot

1 medium diced butternut squash

4 large handfuls spinach

2 tbsp garlic powder

2 tbsp ginger powder

1 tbsp curry powder

1 tbsp turmeric

3 cups vegetable stock

400 ml coconut milk

1 tbsp olive oil

Salt and pepper to taste

Cook onions in the oil until they soften and brown, then add all the spices and garlic and stir well for one minute. Add all the remaining ingredients and bring to the boil. Lower heat and simmer for 20 minutes.

You could multiply the ingredients to make larger batches for the freezer.

Vegetable chilli

(Switch out the sweet potato for turkey or beef mince if you prefer)

2 chopped sweet potatoes

1 large chopped red pepper

1 medium diced onion

2 tbsp garlic powder

3 tbsp tomato paste

400 g can chopped tomatoes

1 tbsp chilli powder

1 tbsp cumin

1 tsp paprika

Salt and pepper to taste

400 g black beans

400 g red kidney beans

Lemon zest

1 tbsp olive oil

Add water as required

Fry onions until they soften and brown. (Add minced turkey or beef at this stage if you are using and fry until browned.) Add tomato paste and garlic and stir together for a minute. Add chopped tomatoes and all the spices and stir well. Add chopped sweet potatoes, peppers and beans and bring to the boil. Simmer for 20 minutes. Add lemon zest, salt and pepper to taste.

Serve on its own with toppings such as sliced avocado, crumbled feta or with quinoa or brown rice.

Energy balls

1 cup rolled oats

½ cup flaxseed or chia seed

½ cup nut butter

2 tbsp cocoa powder

1 tsp honey (optional)

¾ cup medjool dates

2–3 tbsp water

1 tbsp coconut oil

Blend the dates and water to form a paste, then add the other ingredients and mix well into a dough. Use a spoon to scoop and mould into balls and eat fresh or freeze for later.

Alternative snacks

- Freeze dates filled with a nut butter of your choice – slice date in half and add a scoop of nut butter to eat as a fresh snack, or keep a batch in the freezer to have a satisfying and energy boosting snack ready when you need it
- Wholegrain crackers with hummus or yoghurt topped with mixed seeds
- Dark chocolate

9

What to expect after your C-section

Going home from hospital

You've been discharged from the hospital after your C-section and are ready to go home, but that doesn't mean you're ready to resume normal activities. If you'd had any other major surgery, the hospital would likely recommend you rest and take time off from work to recover, so we recommend you treat your C-section recovery in the same way.

The acute healing phase (how long it takes your wound to heal) will last approximately 6–8 weeks, but it's completely normal to still feel pain, numbness and sensitivity for longer. The better you rest and allow healing to occur in those early days, the less likely you are to experience prolonged issues or problems further down the line.

The car ride home

This is often an uncomfortable experience and every tiny bump in the road can feel like a huge pothole that causes pain around your C-section wound. Speak to whoever is driving you home beforehand and encourage them to go as slowly and steadily as is safe, and to consider the route they choose to take home. You may find that bringing a small towel or cushion to place over your scar site in the car and applying a bit of pressure can help limit the pain. Make sure you're dosed up on the pain medication your healthcare provider has recommended before the journey, too.

Rest

The reason you'll see this discussed frequently throughout the book, and it's included early in this chapter, is that it is the most important and best thing you can do for yourself and your wound healing when you get home from hospital. The first two weeks are extremely important for your scar and the more you are able to rest, the better your recovery is likely to be. Delegate chores (or ignore them!), ask for help wherever you can, and definitely stay in bed or on the sofa as much as possible, especially in those first couple of weeks. By following this advice you can help to prevent infections and poor wound healing, both of which can lead to increased scar tissue, infections or pain following your C-section.

Pain

Everyone's pain will be different, so try not to compare your experience to others. Even if you feel great, it's still really important to allow your body to rest and recover in these early days. It really is worth it to give your body and your scar the best possible outcome. You are likely to have been told to use paracetamol and ibuprofen for managing your pain. These medications can work well if taken regularly and as prescribed. They are less effective if taken sporadically. Create yourself a schedule so you can write down and keep track of when and what you have taken to make sure you don't miss a dose or take too many. They may not completely alleviate your pain, but they should make simple tasks like getting up to go to the toilet or move around the house bearable. Please remember that pain serves a purpose to tell you something is wrong, and is usually your body telling you that you need to take more time to rest and recover. If you are taking stronger medication, it could be masking your pain and lead you to falsely believe you are able to do more than you can. This can actually slow or even prevent your healing process from happening effectively.

Expect to feel like even simple things, like getting out of bed and going to the toilet, are going to be a challenge, and put things in place to make this as easy as possible for you (see Chapter 2 on preparing for a C-section).

If you have any concerns that your pain is not manageable, please discuss this with your midwife, OBGYN or family doctor as soon as possible.

Your wound

Your surgeon or nurse will advise you on when to remove your dressing, so make sure you've got this information before leaving hospital. A lot of people find it daunting removing their dressing so if, or when, your midwife visits you at home in the days post-birth, you can ask them to do this for you or taking it off in the shower can help you to feel less fearful. Your wound is likely to be a bit bloody, with crusty scabs along it, you are likely to be swollen around your scar site and through your abdomen. There may be a bit of bruising and redness around it, especially if you had quite a rushed, emergency C-section. The redness may be harder to see on brown and black skin.

Once your dressing is off, it's really important to wash your wound daily with clean water from the shower head, then thoroughly dry it after by gently dabbing it with a clean towel. Once it's completely dry you can get dressed.

Infections

Infections are common after a C-section. Knowing the signs and seeking medical advice as soon as possible is really important to prevent you from becoming seriously unwell. It also helps to ensure the wound heals as quickly as possible to have the best outcome for your scar. Wounds that take a long time to heal and have more trauma in the area (ongoing infections) will create more scar tissue and potentially more issues to your body in the future. We cover what to look out for and how to best care for your scar for a speedy recovery in Chapter 7 on early scar care.

Contact your midwife, OBGYN or family doctor straight away if you have any of the following symptoms after a Caesarean:

- Severe pain
- Leaking urine
- Pain when peeing
- Heavy vaginal bleeding
- Vaginal blood or discharge that smells unpleasant
- Your wound becomes redder, painful and swollen
- Discharge of pus or foul-smelling fluid from your wound

- High temperature
- Feeling faint, dizzy or a fast, pounding heartbeat
- Cough, shortness of breath or chest pain
- Severe headache
- Swelling or pain in your lower leg.

Preventing blood clots

Having a C-section increases your risk of getting a blood clot in your legs, which is called deep vein thrombosis (DVT). As already mentioned, some movement is really important after your operation to help prevent this but if the hospital feels you have a higher chance of getting DVT it's likely they will prescribe you a blood thinning medicine called Heparin too. Your midwife will show you how to inject yourself daily for ten days after your operation. You may need to do this for up to six weeks after if you are at a high risk of developing DVT.

Tell your GP, midwife or health visitor straight away if you have signs of a blood clot, such as:

- A persistent cough
- Shortness of breath
- Swollen or painful lower legs.

Shakes after the birth

Postpartum shakes are quite common after all types of births, but they are more frequent following a C-section and sometimes during your C-section surgery too.

Shivering during the operation is often linked to anxiety or emergency delivery situations. Post-birth shaking, on the other hand, usually occurs because of:

- **Hormonal changes**: The significant hormonal shifts that occur during birth can lower your body temperature.
- **Cold environment**: Operating rooms can be quite cold, and with minimal clothing, it's easy to get chilly.
- **Pain relief medications**: Epidurals and other pain relief drugs can make it harder to regulate your core temperature as they cause blood vessels to expand, increasing blood flow to your skin and resulting in more heat loss.

This shaking typically lasts about 20–30 minutes and can be a bit unsettling. However, rest assured that your medical team is very familiar with this and will provide extra blankets to keep you warm while monitoring your condition. Bringing extra clothes to the hospital can also be helpful. If you know you'll be having a C-section, keeping warm before the operation can make a difference too.

If you experience shaking along with flu-like symptoms, a fever, foul-smelling vaginal bleeding, discharge from your C-section wound, unmanageable abdominal pain, or swelling and redness around your C-section site, please contact your medical team as these may indicate an infection.

Swelling after birth

Due to having a great blood volume, carrying more fluid during pregnancy and the dramatic hormonal change that takes place after delivery in your body, you may notice some swelling. This is common post-birth however you birthed you baby, especially in your feet, legs, hands, face and even your vulva. During a C-section you will also have been given fluids via an IV drip, so alongside these other fluids, this will be dispersed around the body potentially causing swelling.

Try these things to help:

- Drink plenty of fluids to help the body flush out this extra fluid.
- Try to move regularly.
- Elevate your feet above heart level so fluid flows evenly throughout your body and doesn't collect in your extremities.
- Avoid processed and salty foods, which encourage your body to hold on to fluid.
- Wear loose clothing to help improve circulation in your body.
- Try and do short stints of light exercise, such as light walking, to elevate your heart rate slightly and help your body to get rid of the fluid.

Whilst swelling is normal after birth and should go down within a few weeks, it should not be painful. If it is, or you find one side of your body is more swollen than the other, contact your doctor as it could be a sign of a blood clot.

Shoulder tip pain

Something that is often unexpected after a C-section is pain in your shoulder. This is quite common, and is thought to be caused by trapped gas post-surgery putting pressure on your diaphragm muscle, irritating a nerve that then causes pain in the tip of your shoulder. If you suffer with this gentle movement, anti-gas medication and peppermint tea can all help to give you relief. Although this pain can be quite intense, it should subside within a couple of days.

Postpartum night sweats

This is very common amongst new mothers and is a very normal response to hormonal fluctuations that occur during the postpartum period. Your body is getting rid of the additional fluids that were needed during pregnancy. It's more common for it to occur at night, but can happen during the day too. The sweats will usually improve over time and are rarely cause for concern, but if you are noticing that it's really affecting your sleep or you are worried then consult your doctor.

Try to be mindful that more sweating will contribute to dehydration, so it is important to replace fluid lost by staying well hydrated. Hydration is also particularly important for healing and scar tissue formation so you'll need to keep on top of it, and this is even more necessary if you are also breastfeeding.

Good food and hydration

Nutrition should be a big focus after your operation. Water helps to flush out the toxins in your body, reduce swelling, ease constipation and speed up recovery. Lots of protein-rich and nutritionally dense meals will also allow your body to heal quicker; we have lots more information and meal ideas in Chapter 8 on nutrition.

You'll also be advised to drink plenty of fluids to lower your risk of a blood clot.

Clothing

You're not going to want to wear clothing with a waistband that sits on your C-section scar as it will rub and cause irritation. It's best to wear loose fitting clothes made from natural fabrics to allow air to get to the wound and aid healing, and this will be more comfortable if you are experiencing sweats. Get some high-waisted compressive underwear too, as this can really help reduce the swelling and speed up healing. You may want to consider tops that button up the front if you are planning on breastfeeding to save yourself from having to repeatedly lift/untuck tops from your waist to feed, which may also irritate your scar.

Itching after a C-section

Itching is really common after a surgery, and can be caused by a number of factors. It can be really irritating and the urge to scratch is hard to resist, but this will only irritate the area further and potentially cause skin damage and infection. See Chapter 7 on early scar care for how to treat it safely and effectively.

Overhang

This is often one of the main worries of anyone having a C-section. Please know that there are a lot of factors involved here and as such it is often the last thing to go. Our clients often find that their recovery plateaus around ten to 12 months, but it's really important to continue with your rehab and massage; you really can make a big difference and often get rid of an overhang entirely. We have a whole chapter on this (Chapter 23), explaining all the causes and how you can treat them.

Numbness/hypersensitivity

Numbness and hypersensitivity are both really common after a C-section due to the nerves in the area being cut or disrupted during the surgery. These issues can be improved with massage and breathwork, and we cover how to do this in Chapter 24.

Tightness/tension

It's normal to feel tight in the front line of your body immediately after a C-section, and as if you can't stand up completely straight. It's also likely that the scar area will feel tight and restricted. You may also feel nervous about the area and want to lean forwards slightly to protect it and avoid putting any strain on the healing wound. Sleeping in a reclined position with a ramp of pillows behind your head and a pillow under your knees can really help in those early days to make you feel comfortable and less worried. Breathwork and very gentle stretches as you begin to feel better will really help to gently mobilize the scar area and make space through the front line of your body. We cover this in Chapter 26.

Movement

Moving is going to feel difficult. Expect to find even simple things like getting out of bed and going to the toilet a challenge, especially in the first couple of weeks. Put things in place to make this as easy as possible for you (see Chapter 2 on how to prepare for a C-section).

We've already mentioned resting as much as possible in the first two weeks, however mobilizing the scar area a little can help with scar and abdominal recovery. Not only this, but it's likely you'll also hear that it's important to keep active to prevent the risk of blood clots. To clarify, this means doing some gentle bed exercises, pumping your feet and ankles if you're lying or sitting for long periods of time and getting up to move gently around the home at regular intervals to keep your circulation moving. This is VERY different from going out for long walks, doing heavy housework or doing too much lifting and carrying.

For detailed descriptions of the types of movements you should be doing, please refer to Chapter 25.

Mental health

It's common to feel teary or low after birth, often referred to as the 'baby blues'. Changes to your hormones can play a big part in this, and contribute to more extreme highs and lows after birth. If these feelings or emotions continue for more than two weeks after your birth you should seek medical advice as this can be a sign of postpartum depression. If you have been through a particularly traumatic birth or didn't have the birth you planned or hoped for, this can really affect your mood and emotions and can cause long-term psychological problems. Know the signs to look out for and read more about this in Chapter 18 on managing birth trauma.

Some simple tips to help you overcome low mood or negative feelings during early postpartum include:

- Get as much rest as possible and periods of uninterrupted sleep.
- Talk to and connect with other people, both within your family unit and others.
- Try to spend some time outside. When you are physically ready, walking in nature or in the sunshine can help.
- Try to eat healthily.
- Try to get some regular exercise when you are able. This may start with short walks.

Breastfeeding

You may find that laying your baby across you is uncomfortable on your new wound. Using a feeding pillow around your waist is a great way of creating some protection for the scar site. You may also want to investigate alternative feeding positions, such as the rugby hold and side lying position, to avoid pressure over your scar.

Breastfeeding can be very challenging at first, even painful. Usually this improves as you master the technique and your routine becomes more established. When your milk first comes in it can come with a surge of hormones that can make you feel very emotional for a couple of days. When your baby sucks at your breast it stimulates a reaction in the muscles that moves the milk down to the teat, this often comes with a tingling sensation called 'the let-down' which can be very strong and a bit uncomfortable at first.

If you notice your breasts are becoming painful, hot or engorged, or you have a fever alongside flu-like symptoms, you should seek advice from your midwife team or family doctor. These are signs of mastitis, which is common in breastfeeding mothers. It is a condition that can often be self-managed at home, but in some cases will require medical intervention. Seeking support as soon as possible is likely to lead to a quicker resolution and better outcomes.

Your midwife should be able to support you with positioning, latching techniques and help you if you are experiencing ongoing pain that is making your feeding journey hard. Lactation consultants can be really helpful if you are having any feeding difficulties.

Lifting

When you go home after a C-section, you will be told not to lift anything heavier than your baby for the first six weeks. As best you can, this is advice you should take seriously for as long as possible as it prevents excessive strain across your scar, which can result in pulling or tension that affects how it heals.

We know it can be very difficult if you have to carry your baby in a car seat or in their buggy. We also know that many women feel OK before six weeks, and there is often pressure to return to everyday activities including housework, driving or caring for others as soon as possible. Our best advice is to listen to your body, and if you do experience pain with any of these activities, it is a good sign that you are not yet ready. Unless it's absolutely necessary, limit the amount of lifting, pulling and pushing while your wound is healing.

When your scar has closed and you feel ready to be more active or to return to some exercise, we recommend doing some specific postpartum strengthening exercises which will gradually introduce you to lifting in a way that is safe for your scar and postpartum core and pelvic floor. We have written further guidance for introducing exercise in Chapter 20, Chapter 25 and Chapter 26.

Driving after a C-section

Apart from the implications to your recovery, it's likely that your car insurance will also have clauses that will impact your insurance for a period of time after surgery. This is something you should check with your insurance company, as it will be different across the board. Generally the criteria you should consider is whether your scar or pain following your C-section would prevent you from performing an emergency brake manoeuvre if required. For this reason, many consultants recommend waiting at least six weeks before driving.

Tampons

Internal sanitary products are not recommended for use until at least six weeks after birth – it is recommended that you use sanitary pads or period pants instead. This is because you will still have a wound where the placenta was attached to your womb, and it's possible to have cuts or tears in the vagina if you have laboured or attempted an instrumental birth prior to having a C-section delivery. Using internal menstrual products while this is still healing can increase your risk of infection during postpartum bleeding. It is likely that you will bleed heavily in the first couple of weeks after birth, so you'll need to choose products which are suitable.

Your period can return from 4–6 weeks after birth; some people will not have a menstrual bleed for many months or even longer, but others are surprised to find it returns quite quickly. It is not true that you will not have a period if you are breastfeeding. Although if you are exclusively breastfeeding, it is more common for them not to return than for someone who has chosen to bottle feed or partially breastfeed due to the impact on your hormones. It is also possible that your cycle takes a little while to return to its normal pattern. It's recommended you track your periods, as having just one menstrual bleed does not necessarily mean your periods have returned. Many women experience heavier bleeding, more painful cramps and more intense symptoms with the first, or first few, periods following birth. Some women (particularly those who have endometriosis) may notice an easing of symptoms after pregnancy, although this is usually temporary.

Intercourse

Medical advice is to wait six weeks before attempting intercourse after any type of delivery. This is to allow your body to heal, and because of the increased risk of infection. It is possible to get pregnant again even before your menstrual cycle has returned, which is why your 6-week postpartum check-up will often include a conversation about contraception. In the early weeks after birth you may feel sore, still experience bleeding and will likely be very fatigued, all of which can affect your libido, or make sex more uncomfortable. It's important to be aware, though, that it is not normal to find sex painful longer term, and you should seek help if this is the case. Too many women will put up with symptoms because of a lack of information, so please read through Chapter 19 on intercourse after a C-section for a more detailed guide.

Constipation

Constipation and trapped wind are common following a C-section, due to the medication in your system from the operation and because your bowels are moved around during surgery. This affects their normal function and rhythm, and the lack of movement whilst recovering also slows your digestive system and bowel habits. If you are constipated for a long time, it may cause other issues such as pelvic floor problems, haemorrhoids and painful fissures, so it's important to get on top of this as soon as you can.

Things that can help are:

- Gentle movement to stimulate the rhythm of your bowels.
- Drinking plenty of fluids and eating lots of fibre.
- Using a stool for your feet when passing a bowel movement.
- Trying not to strain when having a bowel movement, using your breath to help relax your pelvic floor and gently rocking yourself backwards as you feel the stool moving downwards.
- Gently massaging your abdomen in a clockwise motion.
- Products such as Psyllium husk and lactulose, which you can request from your pharmacist or GP.
- Applying some pressure over your abdomen/scar area with a small rolled up towel to support your wound as you go to the toilet. We've shared a link to a video on this in our 'C-section recovery hacks' in the Resources at the end of the book.

Baths and swimming

The advice on when you can take a bath does vary. Some consultants say you can bathe a few days after, while others recommend waiting four weeks. Generally it's sensible to avoid bathing if your scar is not closing, is very sensitive or irritable or you struggle to dry it properly. Always make sure the bath is clean before filling it, too. You may also find it quite difficult to get in or out of a bath for 3–4 weeks while the tummy is still tender. It's not recommended to wash your wound site with any harsh products or soaps, as this can really irritate and dry out the wound and affect the way the scar develops, so avoid using any bath bubbles or products. Simple rinsing with clean water is best.

Swimming in a swimming pool or in the sea is not recommended until your wound has fully closed and healed and any postpartum bleeding (lochia) should also have stopped, so it's likely to be at least six weeks.

How to cough, sneeze and laugh

These simple movements can be some of the most painful following a C-section, and the best advice here is to support your scar or abdomen first. You could use a pillow or a rolled towel, or otherwise just press your palms over the scar to support the area before you cough or sneeze or laugh. It reduces the pain, feels less scary that your scar or stitches are going to pop open and reduces the amount of pressure on your wound.

Following a C-section birth, you do have to acknowledge that your body may take a little longer to heal due to the nature of surgery and your wound. The scar is naturally going through a lot of change in the first 6–8 weeks and it's especially important in this time that you are not putting any unnecessary strain on the healing tissues or stress on your body.

Postpartum issues you may not be expecting with a C-section

Just because you've had a C-section birth, it doesn't mean you will avoid other postpartum issues that affect the pelvis and pelvic floor. In fact, most often these issues are caused by the pregnancy rather than birth, so it's important that you know what symptoms to be aware of and what to do about them.

Pelvic organ prolapse is very common, affecting around one in three women who have had children. It can affect women after C-section birth or vaginal birth although a C-section birth does decrease the risk. It is usually the result of increased pressure and weight on the pelvic organs and pelvic floor muscles during pregnancy.

Our pelvic organs are supported by a group of muscles and ligaments called the pelvic floor, which also control the bladder and bowel function and help to prevent incontinence. They tolerate an awful lot during pregnancy, as the weight and downward pressure increases as your bump grows. A C-section delivery does not prevent a prolapse from occurring.

You may notice specific activities will make your symptoms feel worse, such as opening your bowels, being on your feet for long periods of time or carrying heavy things. This is simply due to the effect of gravity or fatigue by the end of the day. It's harder for the muscles to hold our organs in place if they also have to work against extra load, such as shopping bags or a heavy baby.

We have included more information in Chapter 18 if you want to find out more.

Pelvic pain is common after pregnancy and birth but is NOT normal. It may be caused by pelvic floor muscles, scars, prolapse, postural changes, spending lots of time sitting/feeding/resting with your baby, or trauma to the coccyx during birth. If you are struggling with pelvic pain, there are lots of things you can do at home to help, or treatments such as physiotherapy to ease your pain. You will find more information about this throughout the book and in Chapter 15.

Leaking after birth – urinary incontinence or bowel incontinence (including passing wind) are common postpartum symptoms. We want everyone to know that while it is common, it is not normal to continue to experience these problems beyond six weeks after birth. Over 80 per cent of women who suffer with urinary incontinence resolve their issues by participating in physio-led pelvic floor therapy.[6]

It's not just leaking that indicates a problem. Other possible bladder or bowel symptoms that can occur after birth include increased frequency or urgency to go to the toilet, feeling that you haven't completely emptied your bladder or bowel, or experiencing pain while urinating or passing a bowel movement.

If you want to know more, read Chapter 15 on recovering your pelvic floor.

This chapter is really a checklist of possible symptoms or concerns that you might experience as you recover from your C-section. We hope that it will ease some of the anxiety you may have and answer some of the questions that often arise during this phase of your recovery. Of course, most of these topics require further explanation to properly understand what is happening to your body. So as you continue to read through the book we'd like to talk you through these issues and provide advice and solutions in the chapters that follow.

My birth story: Hannah

I have always loved hearing and reading about homebirths, so after a long and bumpy fertility journey, which led to IVF and emergency surgery in early pregnancy, I decided to plan for a homebirth. As soon as I met my midwife team, I felt reassured that I had made the right decision.

I really loved being pregnant and tried to stay active whilst also listening to my changing body. I stopped running early on and instead took up swimming, gentle yoga and did lots of walking. I was also fortunate to be able to see Emma in person for a prenatal physio appointment. I found it really helpful to go through some strength exercises and gain a better understanding of how to strengthen my pelvic floor.

The weeks passed by and my due date came and went. I was having reflexology, getting out in nature and doing my best not to get fixated on when our baby would arrive. I had tentatively booked a sweep with my homebirth midwife almost two weeks after my due date. When the day arrived, something felt different, so I asked if I could have reflexology instead. In the early hours of the next morning, my waters broke, and contractions followed.

Four hours later my midwife arrived. My husband had set the birthing pool up, but we decided to continue without it for as long as I could manage. I also had my mum with me, which was so wonderful – she has worked as a doula and was very aware of what I needed without me having to ask.

Once contractions intensified and I began to feel more tired, being in the warm pool was such a relief. After some time, my midwife gave me an internal examination and I was 8 cm dilated, which was reassuring, as I was beginning to worry I wouldn't manage for much longer. After about 15 hours of labouring at home, baby's heart rate began to elevate, and after being monitored for a while, my midwife made the call for us to be transferred to hospital. Despite wanting to birth at home, I knew this decision would not have been made unless my midwife felt it was necessary. The ambulance arrived in minutes, and we were on our way very quickly. Unfortunately for us, there were roadworks and diversions, which meant our journey to hospital took a lot longer than expected. Once we finally arrived, the hospital team were ready and waiting for me. Thankfully baby's heart rate was stable, however I was given another internal examination, which caused my backwaters to break. As a lot of meconium was present, the hospital team strongly advised to proceed with a Caesarean section.

In that moment the most important thing to me was the safety of our baby. I let my birth plan go and put my trust in the medical team around me. Both my husband and I felt quite scared and overwhelmed initially – a few hours earlier we were in the comfort of our own home, which felt calm and relaxed, and now we were heading into theatre surrounded by bright lights and lots of people. Our lovely hospital midwife was so reassuring and kind throughout, explaining what was happening and making sure we were OK. Before we knew it, our little baby girl was passed over the screen; we both cried. She was here and she was safe, in that moment nothing else mattered.

After she had been checked by the paediatrician, we were able to enjoy skin-to-skin, something I had dreamed of. We stayed in hospital overnight and received great care and support from the midwives. I managed to get out of bed the next morning and took a short walk to the bathroom. I felt surprisingly OK (I guess medication and adrenaline were playing a part in that). I was given lots of support with breastfeeding from a wonderful midwife on the ward and, after being given the OK from a doctor, we were discharged. It was a very surreal drive home! I was very grateful to my husband for having been home earlier in the day to clear away the birthing pool and put our living room back together.

The first week or so was a beautiful baby blur. Friends and family sent meals, and my mum did lots of tidying and kept on top of our laundry. I was mindful not to get too carried away with doing lots, but enjoyed getting out in the garden every day.

At about three months postpartum I signed up to The 360 Mama C-section recovery course and began working through it very slowly. I really enjoyed moving my body again with the help of Emma's guidance, and not long after I was able to visit Hannah at her clinic for a scar massage. This was so helpful, and I left feeling much more confident about how to look after my scar.

I am now just over one year postpartum and am still very much adjusting to life as a mum. I am so grateful for all of the help and support from my family and friends, it really does take a village.

10

How long does it take to recover from a C-section?

It takes six months for a scar to fully heal and form and up to two years for it to completely mature (possibly even longer). So you can see why your scar may still be causing you issues months or even years later, particularly if left untreated or with poor wound care at the start.

The acute healing phase (how long it takes your wound to close over and become a scar rather than a wound) will last approximately 6–8 weeks. If your scar isn't closed by this point, book an appointment with your midwife or medical provider to check there isn't something that's preventing it from closing such as an infection. If you have the all clear, then we really recommend following our early scar care information in Chapter 7 and using Medihoney on your wound to speed up healing. Please don't just accept a slow-healing wound as normal, though if this goes on and on, keep going back to your medical provider and push for help to get the wound closed. Often, the longer a wound takes to heal, the more scar tissue you will end up with, and the quality of your scar is often compromised.

It's completely normal to still feel pain, numbness and sensitivity for longer than these initial 6–8 weeks as, although your scar may have formed and your wound closed, your body has a lot of internal healing to do from the surgery you've had. From three months you should feel more like yourself but it's still normal to feel sensitivity, numbness or pain in the area and to feel a weakness through your core. Some people may also feel great after eight weeks post-birth, but it's important to remember that even if you feel fine, your body is still recovering and healing. You still need to build back up slowly to your usual day-to-day routine and exercise schedule to allow your body to heal well and limit internal adhesions.

The better you rest and recover in those early days, the less likely you are to experience prolonged issues or problems later down the line. Have a read of Chapter 7 on early scar care for how to prioritize your healing.

Factors that may affect your recovery

If you had an emergency or unplanned C-section you may have been in labour for hours prior to giving birth via C-section. This could mean your recovery takes a bit longer, as your body is likely to be exhausted and depleted. You may also have had other medical interventions, such as medical induction or attempted assisted delivery with forceps or ventouse, all of which will impact your recovery from birth.

Surgical complications

If your C-section procedure was complicated, it's possible you may have experienced more blood loss than usual during the operation and may find your recovery takes longer. Really focusing on your rest and all the tips we share on optimizing early healing will make a world of difference to how you feel long-term.

Birth trauma

Birth trauma can play a big role in your recovery. If you are struggling after a traumatic birth it's common for your mind and body to hold on to this. You may experience heightened pain and issues in the scar area as well as throughout your body. Massage and introducing touch can make a big difference to this, and physical therapy can help you to accept your scar and support your physical recovery. You will also likely benefit from some specific counselling. We know that physical wellbeing is closely linked with mental wellbeing, and so we recommend addressing both. Please see Chapter 18 for more information.

Pre-existing health conditions

If you have a pre-existing health condition, this can also mean healing is slower and your risk of getting an infection is higher. This is also the case if you:

- Are overweight
- Smoke
- Have diabetes
- Have a poor diet.

Infections

Infections are common after a C-section. Knowing the signs and seeking medical advice as soon as possible is really important. Not only to prevent you getting more seriously unwell, but also to ensure the wound heals as quickly as possible to have the best outcome for your scar. Wounds that take a long time to heal and have more trauma in the area (ongoing infections) will create more scar tissue and potentially cause more issues to your body in the future. We cover what to look out for and how to best care for your scar for a speedy recovery in Chapter 7 on early scar care.

Is C-section recovery harder than vaginal birth recovery?

Every birth is different. We see women who have a C-section and who feel great in themselves in barely any time, and we also see women who birth vaginally who struggle for weeks post-birth to get back to feeling well and more like themselves again. This will all depend on the type of birth you have, how well and fit you are prior to birth, how well the actual birth goes and how well you recover. However, following a C-section birth, you do have to acknowledge that your body may take a little longer to heal due to the nature of surgery and your wound. The scar is naturally going through a lot of change in the first 6–8 weeks, and it's especially important in this time that you are not putting any unnecessary strain on the healing tissues or stress on your body.

Returning to exercise after a C-section

The truth is that returning to exercise after pregnancy and birth however you gave birth to your baby is a very personal journey. It can feel overwhelming with the amount of conflicting advice available about postpartum exercise, especially if you've received an all clear at your 8-week doctor's check but still don't feel right. Our main advice is to listen to your body and if something doesn't feel good, then pause.

We also want to make it very clear that the 'all clear' after your postpartum check-up should not be interpreted as a green light to go back to high-level exercise. As we've discussed above, the acute healing should have happened by 6–8 weeks, but this is just the first phase and your body is by no means back to 'normal' yet. Any exercise should begin gradually, and ideally be supported by a professional who can give you a realistic programme. We know that some people rely heavily on exercise for their mental wellbeing or are desperate to start doing something for themselves after having a baby. But we really recommend not returning to pre-pregnancy exercise before doing some postpartum rehab and strengthening. Not only will this help to prevent injury now, but it will also safeguard you from problems in the future.

It's normal ...

- To still not feel great at six weeks post-birth
- For it to take longer than 12 weeks to get back to 'normal' exercise
- For your tummy to feel numb, sensitive or painful after six weeks
- For your pelvic floor and core to feel weak in the first six weeks after birth
- For you to feel very tired, and for exercise to be the last thing on your mind
- To feel anxious about touching or looking at your scar at first.

It's not normal ...

- To have excessive pain, or for your scar to be weeping, have a foul odour, be very red or hot to touch or to feel feverish
- To be struggling with lots of intrusive thoughts or negative feelings about your birth, which affect your mood or your ability to engage with or care for your scar
- To have bladder or bowel leakage or inability to control wind beyond six weeks after birth
- To feel heaviness or a dragging sensation in your lower tummy or vagina, which worsens with movement or exercise
- To see doming of your abdominal wall when you move, or for your tummy to always look bloated after eight weeks postpartum.

If you do have any concerns about any of these symptoms, do not worry too much. They are all solvable if you know what to look for and seek help with an appropriate professional.

My birth story: Sam

My latest birth story was a delight in comparison to my first. After two miscarriages and a pregnancy during Covid lockdown, I ended up needing an emergency C-section after a failed induction due to premature rupture of membrane. Unfortunately my epidural failed numerous times and they started emergency surgery while I could feel some sensation at the start of the operation. I then had dural migraines that needed a specialist blood patch to fix. All in all, it was incredibly traumatic, I was grateful for my son's safe arrival and for the subsequent counselling and trauma support available afterwards.

Second time round and after further miscarriages we were so thankful to be pregnant again. This time scans showed I had possible placenta previa that may result in another C-section, but it wasn't possible to confirm this until much later in the pregnancy.

Later, when scans confirmed I did not have PP we were offered the option of choosing a VBAC (vaginal delivery after C-section) but we felt so much happier with the idea of an elective C-section. Considering the likelihood of further emergency surgery with a VBAC and the fact both my sons were huge babies, we opted for the C-section.

It was the best decision! Despite the surgery being delayed due to nursing strikes it was a complete breeze. Due to my experience with my previous birth I had a consultant anaesthetist do my spinal and I was shocked at how numb I felt so quickly and without any pain! My second son was born to Classic FM in a beautiful, relaxed moment with skin-to-skin time, he breastfed well and it was just perfect. My recovery was so much better. I was showering and walking around the next morning and going for a walk down the road in a couple of days.

Although sad at the difficulties we have had getting pregnant, the loss of five babies and the trauma from the first birth, we are so grateful to have our children. Our only regret is that the choice of an elective C-section is likely to end our journey of having biological children despite our desire to expand our family.

I am grateful to The 360 Mama for offering such support post C-section where knowledge of rehab is severely lacking.

11

C-section recovery products

There are a number of C-section recovery products on the market to help speed up the healing process of your scar, improve the resulting symptoms and improve the way the scar tissue forms.

Scar tissue is only ever 70 per cent as good quality as 'normal' tissue, which means it's more prone to losing hydration. Wounds need a well-balanced moisture environment to heal well, so adding in a product that not only prevents moisture loss from the wound but adds additional moisture, will both speed up healing and improve the final outcome of the scar.

In the early stages, once your dressing has been removed, it's important to keep your scar hydrated; moisture loss from the area is one of the main causes of poor scar formation. Most oils can't be used until your wound is closed over, but there are some products that are safe to use at an earlier stage.

Medihoney

Can be used on your wound as soon as your dressing comes off. This product is often recommended for scars that have become infected, or are slow to heal and/or have an odour, but all wounds can benefit from using it.

Medihoney is not the same as the honey you find in your kitchen. It's medical-grade Manuka honey, which helps to significantly speed up healing compared to other conventional dressings. It works by:

- Drawing fluid to the surface of the wound, helping to eliminate waste products.
- Creating a moisture-balanced environment, which is best for wound healing.
- Aiding healing with a low PH level and a lower, slightly acidic pH environment.
- Protecting against bacteria, helping to prevent infection.

Medihoney offers a number of products that are available on prescription in the UK from your pharmacist, but which you can also buy online. The ones we recommend are:

- **Medihoney HCS patches**: great for C-sections and can be used from day one. They come in a variety of sizes and can be cut to the correct length if needed. As the patch covers the scar, they provide some protection of the wound against clothes rubbing too. The adhesive ones are easier to use as they are held in place without additional dressings.
- **Medihoney wound gel**: useful if you have a small part of your scar that is still open as you can put the gel into the hole, or if a small section of your wound isn't healing well you can apply it there. This product can also be used from day one.
- **Medihoney barrier cream**: great for use on healed scars (over six weeks old). It can relieve itching, irritated scars, if you're struggling with a rash or thrush in the scar area; this cream is especially good for plus-size clients with an overhang, to aid healing.

Medihoney has a long history of safe use in hospitals. But if you do suspect an infection or are having trouble with a slow-healing wound, please make sure you contact your medical provider first. The brand we recommend doesn't, but other types of medical honey occasionally contain bee venom, so if you have an allergy it's important to check first. Follow the product instructions for how to use Medihoney correctly.

Medical-grade silicone strips

These can improve the outcome of all scars but are ideal for treating hypertrophic (raised) or keloid scars.

Silicone is the top product we recommend to our C-section scar clients. Silicone strips are non-invasive, safe to use and backed by scientific evidence. There are several scientific research studies on using silicone therapy that show it is effective in the treatment and prevention of scars.[7]

By reducing moisture loss from the scar and improving moisture retention, silicone has been shown to:

- Relieve issues such as itching, redness and tension in the scar
- Fade new and old scars

- Help to flatten raised scars
- Prevent scarring from occurring
- Help the scar recover faster.

The strips we recommend also provide full UV protection, which is essential when out in the sun, even if your scar is covered by clothes. On a completely cloudy day, 40 per cent of damaging UV radiation still reaches the earth's surface. Damaged (scarred) skin is more likely to burn and to become permanently discoloured and tighter when exposed to UV rays.

Silicone strips are especially effective in treating **hypertrophic and keloid scars,** and the sooner you use this product the better (although they can be used and have been shown to be beneficial when used on scars of any age).

Silicone can also be applied as a cream or gel but the location of C-section scars means they will be frequently rubbed by clothes, so we find that silicone strips are best for scars in this area. You may want to consider a silicone gel if only a small part of your scar is problematic.

Silicone strips can be used from six weeks post-birth (once your scar is fully closed over and scab free). The one that we recommend is reusable, you just remove the backing on the sticky side and place the strip over your scar, then wash it daily to help it last well and avoid losing its stickiness.

This treatment isn't a quick fix and for best results you need to wear the strip for a minimum of 12 consecutive hours, every day. It can, however, be worn up to 23 hours a day, only removing it to clean the strip and massage your scar.

Rarely, some people find their skin reacts to the silicone and may become irritated. This doesn't mean you can't use the strip, just remove it for a few days to allow the skin to calm down then start the treatment again more gradually, wearing it for an hour longer each day.

You can use oils and creams alongside your silicone strip, but you need to give the cream enough time to soak in before reapplying your silicone strip. Make sure you also only apply your cream/oil to the scar itself and not the surrounding skin, or wipe off any excess oil. Using compression underwear over the top of your silicone strip can help it remain in place better and help it to last longer.

You should expect that the strips we recommend will last you 6–8 weeks and, depending on your scar, you may need to use several kits.

Compression underwear

Compression underwear is beneficial to all scars as it reduces swelling and speeds up healing, but it is especially important if you are prone to hypertrophic or keloid scars.

Supportive high-waisted pants are a must for immediately after C-sections. Not only will they help reduce swelling and speed up the healing process, but the light compression reduces discomfort and protects your wound from rubbing on your clothes. They can also help you to feel less anxious about the area and provide light support to your tummy muscles, helping you to move around more easily.

We recommend buying medical-grade underwear as the weave of the fabric will provide an even pressure across your abdomen that won't stretch over time. This is better for healing and won't cause excessive pressure on your pelvic floor, which can prevent more issues than do good. The fabric will also be moisture-wicking and breathable, which is essential for good healing. Get a few pairs so you can wear them every day.

For keloid or hypertrophic scars, more substantial compression garments are recommended to limit excessive collagen production at the scar site (this is what causes your scar to become raised or keloid) and to support core healing. It is essential that these products are worn correctly, which means they need to fit well, not be too tight or too loose, and that they cover you from your sternum to your pubic bone. For this reason we don't recommend tummy wraps, purely because it's too easy to wear them incorrectly and potentially cause pelvic floor issues due to the compression causing excess downwards force and impacting your pelvic floor function. The compression corset we recommend is medical grade and is designed so that it must be worn in the correct way (as long as you buy it in the correct size.) You will want at least two of these garments so that you can wear them daily.

You can wear compression products from 24 hours post-birth and for as long as you feel you need it but it is recommended to try and have some sort of compression on your scar for the first six months.

Scar-healing creams and oils

These should be used on all scars and are effective at reducing redness, improving tight scars and itching.

Moisture loss from the scar is one of the main causes of poor scar formation, so adding in a scar cream or oil will improve the outcome of your scar. A good scar cream or oil can also help alleviate symptoms such as:

- Itching
- Redness
- Dryness
- Tightness
- Sensitivity.

The main ingredient in a lot of moisturizing products is water (aqua), but water doesn't help alleviate these problems.

The creams and oils that we recommend contain ingredients that have been shown to improve scars such as Aloe vera, jojoba oil, vitamin C and E, rosehip oil, and omega-3 and omega-6 fatty acids. When choosing an oil to put on your scar, try to avoid anything that contains perfumes, fragrance or parabens: these can be detrimental to your healing as they can have a drying effect or may cause sensitivity. Perfumed oils may lead to more itching, redness and irritation and affect the skin's barrier function, impairing the body's ability to retain moisture, which is so important for good scar healing.

For best results use your cream/oil two to three times daily. Some of the oils we recommend can be used as early as two weeks post-surgery but most are recommended for use on scars that have fully closed (around six weeks after birth). It's never too late to improve your scar with these products either. The body's connective tissue is constantly reshaping itself, which is how loosening the adhesions of a scar and improving elasticity is possible even years later.

For how and when to use the specific oils we recommend and how to use the products together, please scan the QR code below.

Product Tutorial

If you're interested in purchasing the products we have talked about here you can find them by scanning the QR code below, as well as some other products that may help your C-section and birth recovery.

12

Breastfeeding following a C-section birth

If you choose to breastfeed, then having a C-section should not be a barrier. There are, however, some things that may impact how your breastfeeding journey starts that could be helpful to know in advance.

If you have an emergency C-section, it's possible that it follows a long and difficult labour, which can leave you feeling exhausted and depleted. Even a planned C-section can leave you feeling exhausted, due to the effects of medication or the impact of having major surgery. This can affect the natural surge of oxytocin that occurs after birth and helps to stimulate your milk supply, and it therefore may take longer for your milk to come in. The best remedy for this is to rest, eat well and give your body the opportunity to replenish its energy stores.

Your body will produce colostrum before your milk comes in, which is a thicker, concentrated food that provides essential nutrients and energy for your baby. It is possible to harvest some colostrum before birth by expressing it from your breasts, usually from approximately 37 weeks pregnant. If your C-section is planned, or even if you hope for a vaginal delivery, it can give you some peace of mind to know that you have a store of colostrum that can sustain your baby while you establish breastfeeding. To reassure you, if you don't harvest any colostrum during pregnancy, you can just hand-express in the hospital to give directly to your baby via a syringe or cup. If you are keen to do this your midwife can advise you how to express and collect it safely before your birth.

Medication

Parents often worry that medications administered throughout the birth, or afterwards will have a negative impact on their baby if it is transferred via breast milk. This is a discussion that is best to have with your medical team, since not all medication protocols will be the same, but typically the risk is very low.

You may have to consider your own ability to feed, depending on your physical state due to the effects of medication. If you are very drowsy, or have had an epidural, which affects your mobility or sensation, then you may need to ask for help when holding or supporting your baby in feeding positions at first. You may have a drip in your arm which could also make it difficult to hold your baby in some positions, or simply feel exhausted after the effort of birth and therefore require some help. There are many positions you can try when trying to achieve a good, deep latch, so it's important to ask for support from someone who has breastfeeding training.

If you find that you are in too much pain from your wound to continue breastfeeding, you can ask your doctor to consider alternative pain medications for a while so that it is more manageable.

Positioning

Skin-to-skin contact is recommended as one of the most important things you can do in the first 24 hours to encourage your baby to latch onto your breast and feed. If you were unable to do this, either because you or your baby were not well enough after birth, it doesn't mean breastfeeding will not be possible, but may take a little longer to happen. Laura Batten, an Infant Feeding Specialist, says, 'In this case, if you are feeling well enough, you can hand-express your colostrum. This could be used to feed your baby, but importantly it will be maintaining your supply. Repeat the hand-expressing as often as your baby would be breastfeeding – so approximately every two to three hours. Once baby is able to latch then there's no need to continue with this pattern of expressing as your baby will be working to keep your supply up instead.'

If your baby is not well enough to feed straight away you may be advised to try expressing some breast milk to encourage your milk to come in. If your wish is to breastfeed, always speak with your birth team so that they can support you to do so.

You may find that one of the difficulties with skin-to-skin contact or feeding after a C-section is finding a position that is comfortable for you and baby. Many typical feeding positions will have the baby resting on your tummy, which could be painful in the early days after surgery because of the pressure on your scar and tummy.

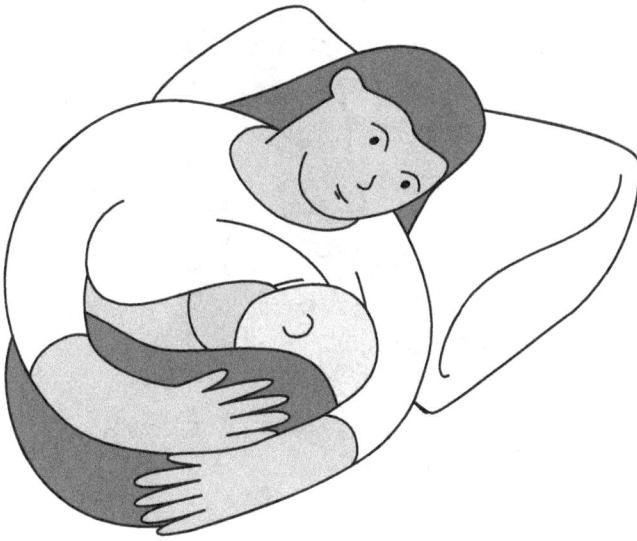

Figure 12.1 Side-lying position for breastfeeding

Some alternative feeding positions to consider are:

- Positioning your baby across you but on some pillows that can protect your incision and reduce pressure on your abdomen.
- Side-lying feeding: lying on your side next to your baby and turning them to face you to latch onto your breast so that there is no pressure on your scar.
- The underarm or football hold, holding your baby to one side with their feet behind your back and neck supported at breast height. Often this can be achieved by positioning your baby on a couple of pillows beside you while you are sitting on the sofa.

If you are using pillows or cushions to support baby, ensure they're able to hinge their head backwards in order to achieve a deep latch.

As your incision heals, your scar will become more tolerant to touch or pressure and feeding will become much easier. Being prepared for the possibility of breastfeeding being challenging at first may allow you to persevere past the initial difficult phase. We'd also recommend you research alternative positions, ask your midwife for advice and support after your birth and let your partner or support network know that they might be expected to help at first. Laura recommends: 'During your pregnancy, research the feeding support in your area: drop-in

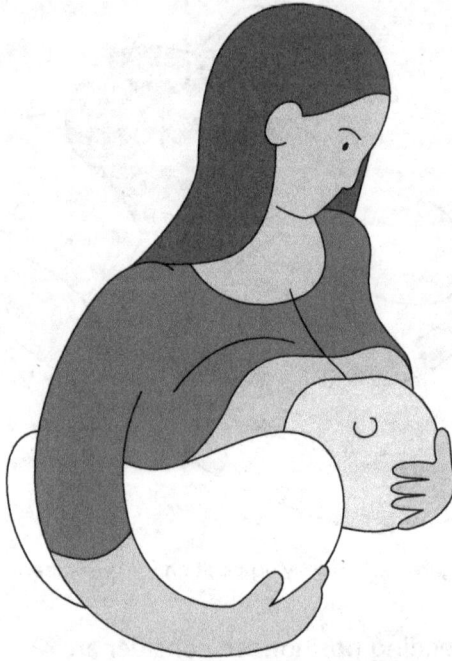

Figure 12.2 Football hold position for breastfeeding

breastfeeding support sessions, IBCLCs, Infant Feeding Coaches or breastfeeding peer supporters. You may experience conflicting advice unless the person supporting you has a qualification in feeding support. With the right help, there's not many breastfeeding issues that can't be supported and resolved with time, care and the right information'.

When to seek help

Breastfeeding can take a lot of time and effort on your part to be successful. A number of factors can affect your journey, and you should always ask for help if you're finding it difficult.

Some babies may struggle with breastfeeding, too, sometimes due to medical issues such as a tongue tie, which may require intervention. Seek a local tongue tie practitioner, ideally one who is also an IBCLC. Some tongue ties won't benefit from a frenulotomy (the dividing of the tie), while others will.

You should also be aware of the signs of an infection or a condition called mastitis that can occur in breastfeeding mothers. It is an inflammation of the mammary gland in the breast, usually caused by a bacterial infection, which can happen if the nipple is damaged. Symptoms include pain; the breast may be swollen, red or hot to touch. You may feel a hard area or lump in the breast caused by a blocked milk duct, or even experience some discharge from your nipple. You may also experience flu-like symptoms or a fever. You should seek medical help in this case as you may require medication. It may be painful to feed if you have an infection, but it is important not to stop feeding suddenly as this can lead to more engorgement and pain. To reduce the inflammation, use ice packs on the breast and lymphatic drainage massage.

Breastfeeding is not an effective method of contraception, so you should continue to take other precautions if you want to avoid another pregnancy.

My birth story: Claire

After five unsuccessful rounds of IVF, I remember the joy of finding out that round number six had, at last, been successful. Being an IVF pregnancy, I had an early scan at 9 weeks at which I learnt that I was pregnant with twins!

It was on that day that the IVF consultant who had guided myself and my husband through our fertility 'journey' said to me, 'get to 37 weeks and have an elective C-section'. At the time that seemed a long way away, but her words stuck with me, and due to the level of trust I had built with her, I kept her advice in my mind while I began to look into twin births.

Of course, everyone's birth stories are different and all are very personal to the person giving birth. For me, and my husband, after the years of longing for a baby and the physical and emotional toll of IVF, we decided that we felt most reassured to choose an elective C-section.

Our NCT group was led by a person who wasn't in favour of what she called a 'cold, sterile' environment for birth, and I can understand that it wouldn't be for everyone. But when it came to our day to have our twins, I remember waddling into the operating theatre and seeing two surgeons, four midwives (two for each baby) with equipment laid out, scrubs on, ready-to-go, and felt an enormous sense of reassurance. Reassurance that this was going to be fine; both babies were going to be fine with experts ready and waiting for their arrival, I would be fine with two surgeons ready to make sure all 3 of us would be in the best possible care.

That's not to say I didn't feel nervous, anxious and a bit overwhelmed, but who doesn't when the time comes to have your baby? But us, after the struggle of getting pregnant, and at times, the fear that it may never happen, it was absolutely the right choice.

Our boys were born within three minutes of each other, and the C-section went without a hitch. If there is one piece of advice I would pass on, it would be that having waddled into hospital at 37 weeks pregnant and having two babies to feed within two hours of being admitted, I had no milk to feed my boys. My milk came in five days after I had them, and we fed them formula and then combination-fed once my milk was available, but I would say to anyone else maybe pack some formula, just in case.

Recovery took a while; six weeks without driving was probably the most frustrating thing. Numbness above and below the incision is still there, but I don't regret our decision at all.

13

What to expect from your postpartum check-up

It's commonly assumed that the postpartum check with your family doctor or OBGYN will include a physical exam and will provide you with all you need to know about how your body has recovered physically from birth. Unfortunately this doesn't always happen.

Following birth, in the UK, the NHS guidelines recommend you will receive a midwife visit at home the day after birth, or on your first day back at home after being discharged from hospital. You should have another midwife visit on day five. You can request further support in the meantime, via a telephone call or additional visits if you or your baby have additional needs. Usually between ten to 28 days after your birth you will be discharged from your hospital midwife team following a final visit. You and your baby will be transferred to the Health Visitor team, who will support you and your baby until they are five years old.

In the USA, it is expected that, once discharged from the hospital, your baby has a check-up three to five days after birth. The ACOG then recommends a check-up for both mother and baby at three weeks.

Currently in the UK, many mothers will either have a telephone consultation or a combined appointment with their baby's first vaccinations when they book their postpartum check-up between 6–8 weeks postpartum. This leaves little, if any, time for a physical examination of your postpartum body, and lots of women report feeling frustrated or let down by the lack of support after giving birth. Similarly, in the USA, not every doctor carries out a physical examination on women and there is a similar gulf between what is needed and what is provided in terms of postpartum care.

You may be surprised to find that not all women will have their C-section wound checked so if you have any concerns about how it is healing, or about infection, ask your health provider to assess it. You should request your midwife look at it during their home visits, or make an appointment to see your doctor any time before the general postpartum check if you have any concerns.

Common signs of poor healing or a wound infection

- Heat
- Redness
- Odour
- Oozing from the site – clear or yellow/green discharge
- Generally feeling unwell in yourself
- Feverish

If you have any of these symptoms, get checked out by your healthcare provider as soon as possible. Infections can cause more problematic scars.

If you are seeing your medical provider but still struggling with a wound that is taking a long time to close or heal, or infection, you may wish to ask your doctor to consider prescribing Medihoney. It is widely used in hospitals and has been shown to be very effective at supporting the wound-healing process. It can be obtained via a prescription but you can also buy this product online yourself. Please see Chapter 11 on C-section recovery products for more details.

It's likely that your doctor will discuss contraception with you during your postpartum check, so it's worth considering what you'd like to do before your appointment. While this can feel premature for many people, do remember that it is a myth that it is not possible to get pregnant again straight away, or while breastfeeding, and so this conversation is important to protect you from another pregnancy while you are still recovering. Additionally, even if you conceived your baby with the support of reproductive technology (through IVF, for example, or while on medication for PCOS), the body does unexpected things post-pregnancy. Previous fertility difficulties are not always an indication that you are still unable to conceive, especially in the early days and weeks following birth. If you are not yet ready to make any decision regarding contraception, you can make an appointment at a later date, but should take other contraceptive measures during intercourse if you want to avoid another pregnancy. Gemma Clifford, a Registered Midwife and Birth Educator in the UK, says, 'It is normally advised to wait 12–24 months post-C-section to get pregnant again, this is because your body needs ample time for healing after such a major surgery. Getting pregnant less than 6 months after giving birth via a Caesarean can increase your risk for a uterine rupture and other complications.'

Your doctor may ask how you are feeling, or ask specific questions about your mental health and your relationships at home during this appointment. If you are struggling with your mental health, feel low or have noticed changes with your mood, then ask for specific help. It can feel difficult to open up, or you may just be waiting for these feelings to pass, but seeking support early on can make a big difference. You can also find out about other local support groups, places to socialize with other new mothers or more formal mental wellbeing services in your area. Postpartum depression can include having negative feelings and thoughts about your birth, and birth trauma counselling can really help with this.

You may find the guest blog on our website from an NHS GP about understanding postpartum depression helpful.

the360mama.com/blogs/understanding-postnatal-depression-from-a-gp-perspective

If you're worried about having this conversation with your doctor, below are some helpful topics you could consider to begin with. Use the page to add your own notes so you can take them with you to your appointment. It's easy to forget what you wanted to talk about on the day, especially if you are tired from or distracted by caring for your baby.

Topics to consider for your postpartum check-up

- Are you getting any periods of quality sleep? Can you rest during the day? Can you sleep when your baby sleeps? Do you have anyone who can help when you need to rest?
- How often are you feeling tearful?
- How much support do you have at home?
- Are you feeling fearful or anxious? How often? Are there any recurring triggers or thoughts?
- Are you socializing with or without your baby at all?
- Do you have negative thoughts or feelings about your birth experience?
- What support or treatment options are available for me?
- Is it safe for you to take medication if necessary? How would your doctor decide whether this was the right option for you?
- Other worries or concerns

_____

_____

_____

_____

_____

_____

_____

_____

_____

_____

_____

_____

_____

See Chapter 18 on managing birth trauma for more specific advice and information about dealing with birth trauma and how to seek help.

In the UK, the NHS also offers a post-birth service called Birth Stories. It gives you the opportunity to discuss your birth experience with a midwife and understand why certain decisions were made during your birth. This can help you to process the outcome of your birth, allow you to feel better prepared or informed should you decide to have another baby in the future, or just give you the opportunity to ask any questions you may have.

If you do not receive a physical check-up, then please do not assume that you are ready to return to exercise just because you've hit the 6-week mark. While 6–8 weeks is the estimated average time for tissue to heal from acute trauma, it is very unlikely it is ready to be under significant strain or withstand much force. To recover properly, you will need to follow a rehabilitation programme, which will introduce you to exercise and movement in a way that supports your recovery rather than overdoing it. Following a C-section, you'll need to consider how pregnancy has affected your body as well as the birth itself. Your scar will often still be changing and healing a lot internally, even when it looks healed from the outside.

Whenever you choose to start exercising again, remember it's important to start from scratch and build up your tolerance, strength and fitness slowly so as to avoid injury or problems later on. It is necessary to take into consideration the changes your body has gone through, and while you might feel good, it's very unlikely you'll be able to return to the same level of exercise post-pregnancy straight away. It is often our experience that family doctors and even OBGYNs are not able to offer much advice in regards to the safety of exercise in postpartum, and we do encourage you to seek an assessment from a physiotherapist/physical therapist who specializes in that area of expertise.

Your postpartum bleeding (lochia) should stop by approximately six weeks. It can stop and start during this time, but if you are still bleeding after six weeks, or if you are experiencing heavy bleeding after the first few weeks, or if it smells unusual, then you should ask your doctor to assess you. If you have experienced heavy blood loss during or after your birth you may wish to ask your doctor to do a blood test to check your iron levels and make a decision whether you would benefit from taking any supplements to aid your recovery.

These are some questions that you might want to prepare prior to attending your appointment for your doctor.

Questions to ask at your postpartum check-up

- Can you check my C-section scar for signs of infection or to check that it is healing well?
- Can you check for signs of diastasis recti (abdominal separation)? (Ask for a referral to a Women's Health Physiotherapist if you do have signs of diastasis recti)
- Ask for an internal check for signs of prolapse if you have symptoms or concerns. (Ask for a referral to a Women's Health Physiotherapist if you do have signs of prolapse)
- Ask for medication or advice to help manage constipation as straining is not good for pelvic floor recovery
- Ask for a referral to physiotherapy/a physical therapist if you are still experiencing incontinence (either urinary or bowel)
- Ask for support if you are finding sex is painful since giving birth
- Can you prescribe or suggest anything to help with vaginal dryness or discomfort? (This is particularly common when breastfeeding and is due to hormonal fluctuations during early postpartum).
- Ask for an assessment of your breasts if you are having trouble with breastfeeding, experiencing pain in one or both breasts, noticing lumps or blocked milk ducts or feeling feverish or unwell. Mastitis can develop as a result of blocked milk ducts when breastfeeding. You may be able to ask for a referral to a lactation support service, which can be really beneficial both in preventing the onset of mastitis or managing it.
- If you are in the UK, and want to discuss your birth experience with a midwife or birth team, ask to be referred to Birth Stories.
- If you have experienced heavy blood loss, ask for a blood test to check your iron levels
- Ask for support for your mental health if you are struggling.

_____

Being prepared for your appointment means you can advocate for yourself and your needs better, but sometimes due to a lack of referral options or resources you may have to consider self-funding for access to private specialists. Again, this is a personal decision and may not always be possible, but it is still important to know what services do exist so you can make an informed decision about the best care for you and your baby.

My birth story: Whitney

In 'America is Failing its Black Mothers', an article written by Amy Roeder in the _Harvard Public Health Magazine_, Amy writes:

'The CDC now estimates that 700 to 900 new and expectant mothers die in the U.S. each year, and an additional 500,000 women experience life-threatening postpartum complications. More than half of these deaths and near deaths are from preventable causes, and a disproportionate number of the women suffering are black.'

Throughout my entire pregnancy, my health was top-notch. It wasn't until my boyfriend and I went to the maternity unit to prepare for birth that the nerves started to rise.

I was in the hospital at 39 weeks and three days. Unfortunately, my son's heartbeat would drop now and then. I also wasn't dilated enough, so they inserted a balloon to help quicken dilation. My night there was uncomfortable. I kept waking up in the middle of the night because of the pain and heard what seemed to be someone in intense labor next door. The noise amplified my anxiety, and I became nauseous. So much so that a nurse prepped a needle without my consent to ease nausea. Thanks to #pregnancytok, I remembered one of my rights as a pregnant woman: the ability to speak up and deny certain practices if you do not want them.

After a day, an intern checked how many centimeters I was dilated and was excited to hear I was at 7 cm; active labor! As the contractions and pain increased, I gave in to having an epidural. You would think I would get ready to push once my doctor came back into the room. Nope! I felt my anger meter go up when I discovered I wasn't at 7 cm but stuck at 4 cm. It was a human error.

A few more hours went by, and I had to get rushed into an emergency C-section. A swarm of doctors surrounded me and flipped me to try to hear my son's heartbeat. My boyfriend and I immediately became nervous, and I started vomiting.

Immediately tears started flowing down my face. I couldn't stop crying and couldn't see the one person who could console me; my boyfriend. However, during that brief absence, an anesthesiologist tried to calm me by passing his latex-dressed hand over my head, but he was a stranger to me, and at that moment, I had no trust in doctors.

A familiar voice came to my side, holding my hand, saying, 'Baby, he's here ... do you hear him?' I slightly heard my son's cries, but I mainly felt doctors tugging at my skin and accommodating my biological structure. A pale baby hovered over the side of my face, and I felt some relief and joy. It was over.

It was 1 a.m. when I got to look at him, make my first attempt at breastfeeding him, and kiss him. *'Eso fue un arroz con mango,'* as my Afro-Cuban mother would say. 'That was a mess.'

Days later, after extremely painfully swollen feet, an inability to inhale correctly, and chills, I ended up in the hospital – one in a different location.

I was later diagnosed with pre-eclampsia and ended up in the high-risk unit. But, again, I had no clue what that was. I cried intensely because between the sleepless nights, the discomfort, and the multiple emotions running through my mind, I couldn't comprehend what the doctor was trying to explain.

I had spent two days in the high-risk unit. I mostly slept those days and had visits from my mom and boyfriend, though slight depression started to creep in because I couldn't take care of my son.

When I finally left the hospital again, I was a different person. I find myself trying to catalog the timeline, reliving the minutiae during my day-to-day activities of what had happened. Although constant efforts are underway to improve maternal health, according to the Black Maternal Health Caucus, I can't seem to get over the traumatizing sequence of events, constantly plagued with questions. Why is maternal health, let alone black and brown maternal health, ignored? Why don't some doctors inform black and brown patients about health risks to be wary of? Who stands up for us?

The 360 Mama: *As we write this book, we are aware of the alarming statistics from both the UK and the USA that highlight the discrimination that women of colour experience throughout their maternal care. Whitney's story is an important one, and we are grateful to her for sharing it in the hope that it might help others advocate better for themselves and raise awareness for the campaigns to improve maternal healthcare for Black and Brown women across the world. Below are some helpful resources that we'd like to share with you if this story has affected you, or you are navigating your own journey.*

USA

https://blackmamasmatter.org/

https://blackmaternalhealthcaucus-underwood.house.gov/

UK

https://fivexmore.org/

14

Diastasis recti (tummy muscle separation)

Diastasis recti refers to the separation of the abdominal muscles, usually as a result of pregnancy and childbirth. It's often a cause of some concern for women during the postpartum period because it can affect the appearance of your midsection, contribute to discomfort or feelings of weakness in the core, or cause abdominal or back pain. It may also impact when you can return to exercise, and what type of exercise is appropriate for you as you recover from pregnancy and birth.

A typical presentation of diastasis recti is a bulging or coning appearance along the midline of your tummy while there is pressure in the abdomen, such as might occur when you are sitting up from a lying position or lifting something heavy. Some women describe themselves as 'still looking pregnant' months after childbirth, as the abdominal wall has not returned to its previous shape or position.

It may help to point out that the gap is a normal part of pregnancy and will affect 100 per cent of mothers beyond 35 weeks of pregnancy. It is necessary for the two sides of the abdomen to move in order to accommodate your growing bump and baby. Rather than imagining the muscles 'splitting' it is actually the connective tissue that bridges the gap between the left and right side of the tummy muscles stretching and thinning. This connective tissue is called your Linea Alba and runs from the breastbone to the pubic bone between the tummy muscles called *rectus abdominis* or the 'six pack'. It might help to identify it as mirroring the dark line that appears on your pregnancy bump. The separation, or gap, can be the full length of the abdomen, or it may occur in just one area.

This bridge of connective tissue, alongside the muscles, helps to form a continuous wall across the abdomen that can withstand pressure and provide support. If this structure is significantly stretched and therefore thin, as in the case of diastasis, it can become vulnerable when under pressure. Imagine a piece of cling film and then imagine pulling and stretching the film apart in the middle. To look at the piece now, you'd

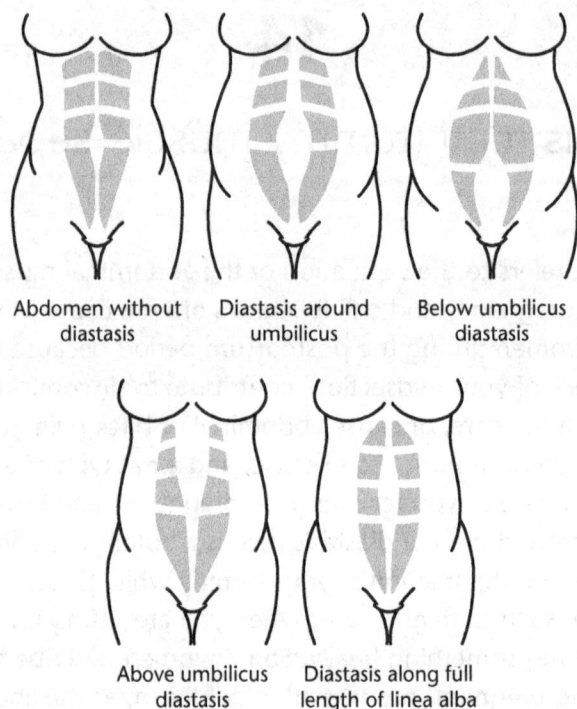

Abdomen without diastasis   Diastasis around umbilicus   Below umbilicus diastasis

Above umbilicus diastasis   Diastasis along full length of linea alba

Figure 14.1 Different types of diastasis

be able to see the area that you've stretched as it would have a different appearance, and the cling film would have altered in shape and be thinner in the stretched spot. It would be easier to tear it in that place than in part of the film that has not been touched or altered.

Some possible outcomes of a poorly managed diastasis include:

- Umbilical hernia
- Abdominal pain
- Bloating
- Pelvic organ prolapse
- Urinary or bowel incontinence
- Constipation
- Back pain
- Painful sex
- Swollen/protruding abdomen.

Evidence is still limited to explain why some women will notice the diastasis gap close within 6–12 weeks, while others will not. It is likely that there are numerous contributing factors, different for everyone. Some common influencing factors include:

- Posture: One example of this would be if you were regularly slouching or rounding your shoulders or slumping in a chair, which is very common for a mother feeding/carrying/cuddling baby. You may be compressing the upper abdomen and creating pressure in the lower abdomen, causing it to 'bulge' against the thinner connective tissue.
- Breathing patterns: Diaphragmatic breathing is a way of breathing that requires you to breathe in deeply through the nose and out through the mouth. It encourages the diaphragm, a muscle that sits under the lungs and above the abdomen, to rise and fall and improves lung function. The tummy and the chest should inflate as you breathe in and expand, and fall as you breathe out. This type of breathing encourages a natural expansion and flattening of the tummy as the core and pelvic floor muscles work in synchronization. Pregnancy can often change our breathing patterns and habits, meaning that the core does not function as well.

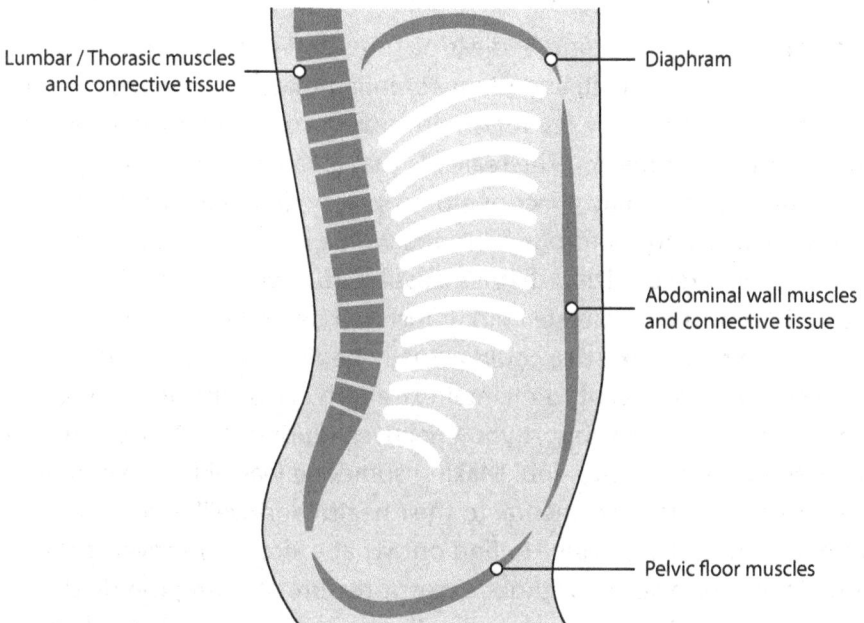

Lumbar / Thorasic muscles and connective tissue

Diaphram

Abdominal wall muscles and connective tissue

Pelvic floor muscles

Figure 14.2 The pelvic floor

- Movement patterns: For example if you have a habit of bracing the tummy, or holding in your tummy, very tight muscles on the side of your abdomen or weak abdominal and pelvic floor muscles, you may make compensations in the way you use your body.
- Previous history of connective tissue disorders (such as Ehlers Danlos syndrome, Marfan Syndrome or joint hypermobility syndrome): If the connective tissue is already prone to overstretching or you have a collagen defect, it is likely that the linea alba will be similarly affected as a result of stretching through pregnancy.
- Scar tissue from a C-section scar can also cause pulling of the surrounding tissue towards the scar line or to one side which makes it more difficult for the abdominal muscles to come back together uniformly.
- The more pregnancies you have, the more times the connective tissue will change and stretch, so midline separation is more likely to occur. This is also true for twin or multiple pregnancies as the abdominal tissue is likely to stretch more.
- Age may also be a factor in how well your tissue heals and repairs, the amount of collagen available, and if you have pregnancies very close together as the tissue has less time to repair in between.

Look online and you'll find endless pictures and posts about the dangers of diastasis recti and plenty of inflammatory language causing women to become very fearful of movement – particularly of exercises such as sit ups or planks. The reality is that it can present in many different ways and may affect one person very differently from another, so it's unhelpful to try to put everyone with a diastasis in one box.

We're now recognizing that it's possible to have a 'functional diastasis' which can tolerate load, effort and be challenged. In this scenario, avoiding exercise could actually be detrimental to your recovery since you want to maintain strength across the abdominal wall to ensure it can support you effectively during day to day activities. Motherhood is a physical job! Making someone fearful of movement and exercise is also detrimental to their health and wellbeing in the longer term. It is important to find out what exercise or movements you can perform safely, without excess pressure affecting the diastasis. Some people will cope really well with one movement, while others would do better in a different one, so getting a personal assessment is always recommended. This allows you to begin to exercise sooner, work on the areas that are most beneficial for you and regain your confidence and strength again.

Even those people who have a dysfunctional diastasis will need to address it with exercise that challenges them to a level that is right for them. It may be that this begins with simple breathwork, it might require modified versions of exercises or it might include challenging workouts – but it's a form of rehabilitative exercise that is specifically targeting their dysfunction. With the right support, diastasis is usually very responsive to rehabilitation and most women will eventually be able to return to their chosen sport or exercise without barriers.

In some extreme cases surgical correction of diastasis may be offered, which involves a repair of the gap, bringing the two sides of the abdominal muscles together. This can help to improve core function and support and improve the appearance of the tummy, which often bulges or protrudes as a result of the diastasis. While some women may seek out surgical options because they are unhappy with how their tummy looks, it's worth considering whether it causes you any physical symptoms first. It's a very invasive surgery, will leave you with a considerable scar and scar tissue and will require extensive rehabilitation afterwards. Similar to our advice surrounding C-section recovery, we'd recommend doing plenty of research beforehand, finding health professionals who can support you through the process and making adequate plans for your recovery if you feel that correction surgery is right for you.

In short, it is essential that women receive the right education and information to allow them to seek appropriate advice, treatment and training. The optimal level of assessment is from a women's health specialist physio. They will be able to: assess your abdominal separation, how this changes and works during movement, how this affects your posture and movement, what effect breathwork makes to your degree of separation or midline control, and how the connection between your diaphragm, abdominals and pelvic floor muscles behave.

Specialist physiotherapists are unique in their ability to assess the pelvic floor function both externally and internally, alongside a full body movement screening after birth, giving the client so much more information about why the diastasis is not recovering or not functional. While it may be a common outcome of pregnancy, it's not necessarily something you have to live with, and certainly not if it's affecting your quality of life or ability to stay fit and healthy. If you have concerns regarding diastasis following pregnancy, or you recognize some of the symptoms mentioned above, seek an assessment with a women's health physio. Understanding your condition and how it affects your body will enable you to train effectively, achieve better results and gain body confidence.

My birth story

My contractions started on 26 July 2023 in the middle of the night. They were on and off and not consistent. By 6 a.m. on 27 July they had stopped, and didn't start again until 5 p.m. on 27 July. I'd lost my 'bloody show' and the contractions were on and off from there onwards. Sometimes I'd have contractions every three minutes and then not for ten minutes. Sometimes my contractions would last up to three minutes, which was extremely painful.

I went through the initial contractions on my own because my partner was working nights. I used an app to help with breathing techniques. Midday on 28 July I was starting to worry about the 'bloody show' because it didn't stop, and worried that my contractions were lasting so long. I rang the hospital and they confirmed to me that everything was normal and they advised me to have a bath to help me feel more comfortable and to try to reduce stress. Between midday and 4 p.m. I rang the hospital another two times because I just felt like something wasn't right. This was my first pregnancy and despite having completed antenatal classes, I felt out of my comfort zone and I was starting to struggle with the pain. Paracetamol was not cutting it.

I was invited in for an assessment on the labour ward, fully expecting to be sent home. When I arrived at the hospital I had only dilated 2 cm, but my blood pressure was sky high, which meant I was not allowed to go home because they had concerns of pre-eclampsia, despite no other symptoms or history of blood pressure issues. I was given some medication to help bring down my blood pressure. At this point consultants came into the room to discuss my options, and I had to go onto the hormonal drip. I wasn't allowed a C-section at this point due to concerns that my blood pressure was high and could cause a lot of blood loss.

Because I was speaking to consultants and midwives, my contractions had completely stopped. I begged the consultant to allow me to try and go into labour naturally, because I really didn't want any medical intervention. They gave me two hours. I walked up and down the stairs of the hospital and around the hospital grounds. My contractions had started again and felt a lot stronger. When I got back to the room I was given gas and air to help. When I was assessed again, I hadn't dilated any further and my waters had broken, so I was advised that they needed to speed up the labour. I asked for an epidural at this point because I knew from my antenatal classes that the hormone drip would be very intense, and I was already struggling with the pain.

I had to wait until 2 a.m. on 29 July because the anaesthetist was coming in from a different area and was stuck in theatre. The epidural was really straightforward and worked instantly. At this point I was able to relax and get a little rest. At the point of the first check, after the drip had been in for approximately eight hours, I had only dilated 1 cm. I was so disheartened, but begged the consultant and midwife to allow me another two hours to see if I would progress anymore. I was so adamant that I wanted a natural birth but in all honesty, looking back I don't know why I fought it so much because by this point I was exhausted.

Another two hours later I'd progressed to 4 cm dilated, but the baby's heart rate was dropping. It was decided a Cat 2 C-section was the best step to take in order to protect the baby's life and mine. I burst into tears when I was told this. I was exhausted, relieved that it would be over soon, but also so terrified. I'd never had surgery in my life and had visions of me being on the table being cut up and the pain relief not working. My midwife completely reassured me and discussed the process with me. The anaesthetist also came to see me and discussed the procedure with me. When in theatre all the staff were really friendly, and the anaesthetist stood by my side for the entire procedure. He ensured several times that I could not feel anything below my ribs, so that I was confident I'd be safe. He kept reassuring me throughout the surgery and kept me calm.

The screen went up and within a matter of minutes my baby was born, on 29 July 2023 at 4.16 p.m. weighing 7 lb 7 oz. My baby was wrapped up in a towel and brought straight to my side so I could say hello. She was then taken to be weighed and my partner cut the cord. I think the whole procedure lasted approximately an hour. It was really straightforward and there was no need for me to be worried. I was really well looked after and my scar is very neat.

In terms of recovery, the first week was really difficult. I was in pain, and it was difficult to move about. I felt very debilitated. On Thursday 3 August, I managed a small walk outside with my husband and baby in the pram. From there on, I made sure I walked a little every day, increasing the distance when I felt comfortable too. It was very noticeable when I had done too much, because the scar area would swell a little, or bleeding would increase. Before pregnancy I was a fit and healthy woman. I went to the gym at least three or four times a week and I think this helped with my recovery. Four weeks in, I felt almost back to normal, but continued to take it steady and didn't return to exercise until 13 weeks postpartum due to abdominal separation (diastasis).

We are hoping to have a second baby in the next few years, and I am contemplating whether to elect for a C-section due to the issues we had above and to ensure safe delivery of the baby.

15

Recover your pelvic floor

Many women believe that because they've had a C-section birth, they'll avoid the other postpartum issues that affect the pelvis and pelvic floor. In fact, often these issues are caused by the pregnancy rather than by birth so it's important that you know what symptoms to be aware of, and what to do about them.

In the case of an emergency C-section, delivery often follows several stages of labour, so your body has to recover from this effort, as well as heal from surgery. This can be particularly impactful on your pelvic floor, and should be considered when you are thinking about your recovery.

Please also bear in mind that you don't have to be experiencing symptoms to include pelvic floor recovery in your postpartum plan. **All pregnancies will place significant strain on the pelvic floor muscles, and all pelvic floors will benefit from rehabilitation post-birth.** This is another reason why resting in the first days after birth is recommended, to reduce the strain on the muscles when they are vulnerable. Offloading them for a few days while you rest in bed gives them the opportunity to properly recover and can make a real difference to how you feel down below when you do start moving again.

Typical symptoms caused by a pelvic floor that hasn't properly recovered include feeling heavy or achy in your pelvis or genital area, leaking urine or faeces, struggling to hold wind, or feeling pressure or a bulge in your vagina. Often these feel worse when you are upright, standing, or after physical activity such as walking or lifting your baby.

What is the pelvic floor?

The pelvic floor is a group of muscles that are located within the pelvis, between the tailbone at the back and pubic bone at the front. They provide support for the pelvic organs, the bladder, bowel, uterus and vagina in women, and prevent urinary or bowel incontinence. Alongside this function, they are also important for sexual function and pleasure.

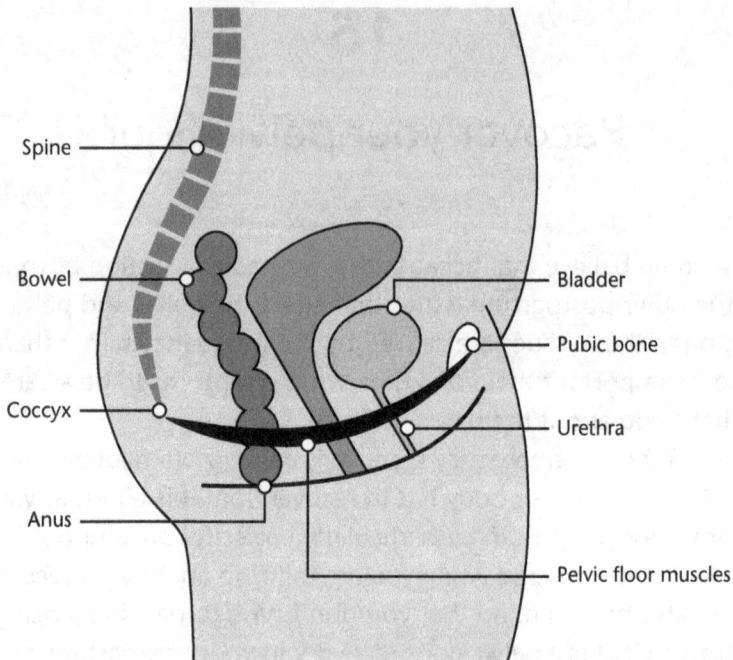

Figure 15.1 The pelvic floor 'sling'

You can imagine these muscles as a hammock that cradles the pelvic organs, lifting them when required and providing support from below when they are under strain.

When you squeeze or contract your pelvic floor muscles they lift and tighten, helping to lift the organs above it, while the circular bands of muscle that surround the opening of the urethra, vagina and anus squeeze shut, stopping the flow of urine, faeces or wind. If you look at the image of the pelvic floor below, you'll notice that most of the muscles have attachments to the back end of the pelvis, so you are likely to feel a more effective squeeze and lift if you visualize lifting from the back towards the front. Helpful visualizations can include stopping yourself from passing wind followed by stopping the flow of urine, pulling a zipper closed from the tailbone to the pubic bone, or lifting a tampon higher into the vagina.

(You should note here that it is NOT recommended to ever practise stopping the flow of urine while actually passing urine on the toilet as this can increase the risk of urinary tract infections (UTI).

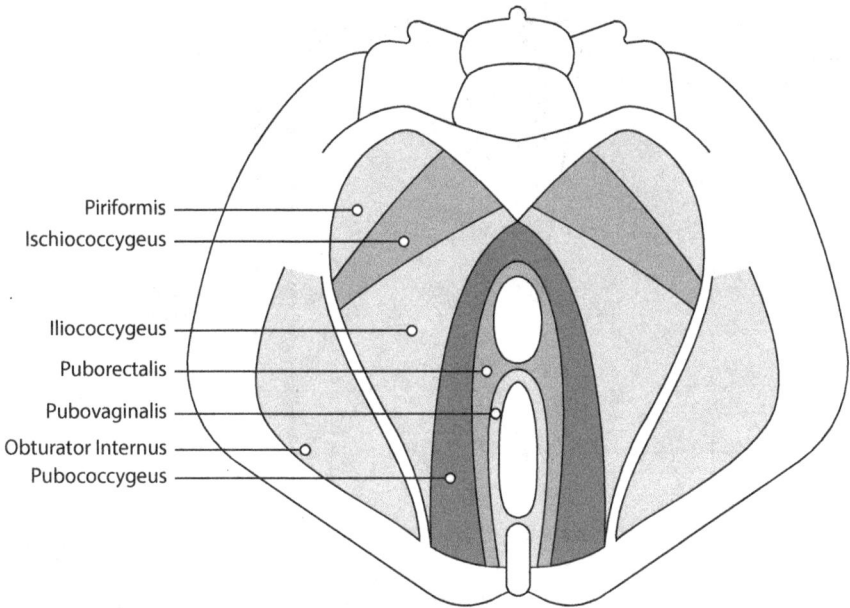

Figure 15.2 The pelvic floor is made up of more than one muscle

Because of the connection between the diaphragm and the pelvic floor muscles, it is helpful to imagine them as a pair, with the diaphragm stacked directly above the pelvic floor. For them both to work effectively they need to mimic each other's movement at the same time. This is why breathing exercises are such useful postpartum exercises that you can begin straight away.

Taking a breath in (inhaling) requires the diaphragm to flatten and move downwards to allow for the lungs to expand as they fill with air. As you breathe out (exhaling), the diaphragm lifts and contracts to help push the air out of the lungs. Now, consider the pelvic floor muscles mimicking this. It means that as you are breathing in, the pelvic floor muscles are lengthening, relaxing and moving downwards, and as you breathe out, they lift and contract. So when you want to perform pelvic floor exercises, to achieve a powerful and effective lift and contraction (or the squeeze in a kegel – an exercise aimed at improving the strength of the pelvic floor muscles by performing a squeeze and a release of the muscles), it needs to be performed during an exhale.

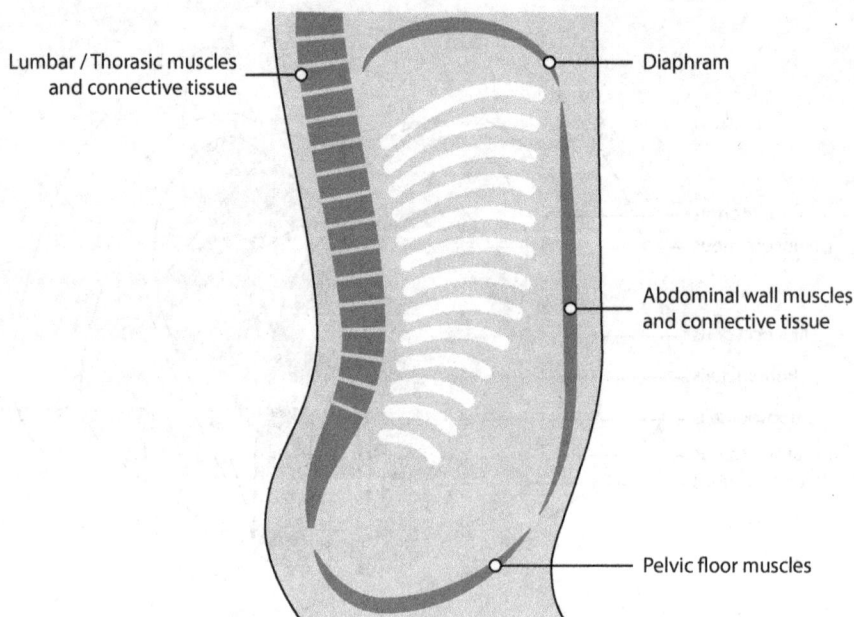

Figure 15.3 The diaphragm / pelvic floor stack

Often just making this small change to your exercises will make a big difference to how you feel when you're practising your kegels. It's also really important to always take a full breath in between efforts to allow the pelvic floor muscles to fully let go and relax before you repeat the next squeeze. Think of doing bicep curls at the gym, you need to squeeze the bicep to lift the weight, and then let it go to straighten the arm back out again before you go again. It's an important part of the exercise.

Once you've mastered the technique of effectively squeezing and letting go of the pelvic floor muscles, you can start to introduce more challenging exercises to your routine.

Video: Pelvic Floor Muscle Training Tutorial #1

To follow video instructions of the exercises that follow in this chapter, please use the QR code to visit our physio-led exercise library.

https://www.youtube.com/@the360mama/videos

We recommend starting your pelvic floor exercises in a lying position or in child's pose because the pelvic floor muscles are easier to connect with. This is because we are removing the load of gravity, body weight and the impact that our posture can have on these muscles. You should be able to feel the squeeze and the release when you perform the exercises. Aim to do ten repetitions of a lift and squeeze as you exhale, and a full release as you inhale. For now, work at your own pace. This is the start of reconnecting with the pelvic floor muscles again. The body and brain are very good at making compensations when we get into bad habits, or we sustain an injury, or when pregnancy alters the way in which we move. It is likely that following pregnancy you will struggle to find a connection with the pelvic floor muscles at first, but with regular practice you can get the brain and body feeling more in sync, and eventually encourage the pelvic floor muscles to work more automatically.

When you have mastered this, try to also include holding the squeeze at the top of your range for ten seconds, followed by a full release as you inhale. You should aim to repeat this ten times. This will help to build endurance and control, meaning the pelvic floor can work effectively throughout the day or during activity when they may tire.

The pelvic floor also has to be able to react to a sudden movement, or change in pressure such as what happens when we cough, sneeze or jump. For this function to improve, you will also need to introduce faster repetitions of the exercises we've described above. We recommend working through the earlier steps first, since it is often harder to perform the faster repetitions and you'll benefit from having 'reconnected' with the muscles first. When you do perform them, be mindful of allowing the muscles to still fully let go between squeezes – this is often what most people struggle with at first. To cope with the sudden change in pressure the muscles will need to first lengthen and absorb the force, before then springing back to squeeze, lift and support (think of how a trampoline works). If the muscles can't move efficiently in both directions, this may be why you're experiencing leaking or discomfort.

Individual muscles within the pelvic floor attach to different sites. These include the sacrum, sitting bones, coccyx and sides of the pelvis. This means the pelvic floor muscles can contribute to pain in the hips, tailbone, lower back and abdomen – all areas in which new mothers will complain of pain in pregnancy and after birth. They also make up part of the core system, which includes your deep abdominal muscles, back muscles and diaphragm, which act as a team to support and give strength to your mid-section. Since pregnancy can put considerable pressure on this area of the body, it is very common to feel lacking in core strength postpartum, or to suffer the effects of a poorly functioning core. Trying to build greater core strength, while only focusing on the abdominal muscles, is unlikely to be very effective, as we require the whole system to work effectively to achieve good core strength. This is another (and often overlooked) reason to include pelvic floor exercises as you recover from birth.

Understanding the anatomy of the muscles also helps to explain why the pelvic floor can be responsible for back pain, tailbone pain, hip pain, pelvic pain or deep abdominal pain. Often in these cases, repetitive kegels or 'squeezing' is likely to make the pain worse. Imagine clenching your fist tightly all day; it's likely to feel very stiff and achy after a while, and eventually the fingers, hand, wrist and even elbow would start to hurt. The same theory applies to the pelvic floor, and yet it is very common to find that people struggle to relax their pelvic floor muscles. This can be influenced by many external factors, too. Some examples include the belief that a 'tight' pelvic floor is good; dealing with birth trauma, or struggling with events surrounding your pregnancy or birth that means the pelvic floor is in protective mode; symptoms of bladder or bowel issues that leave you feeling nervous to relax the pelvic floor for fear of leaking, historical sexual abuse or experiences, and sometimes in athletic populations, (particularly dancers and gymnasts) where holding in the core is encouraged. You may also identify with the idea of 'holding tension in the body' or have experienced tension headaches, clenching your jaw or grinding your teeth when you are stressed or anxious. This is often a good indicator of whether your pelvic floor muscles may behave in a similar way, and so it's important that you master the technique of releasing the muscles, as well as being able to squeeze them.

Ideally, you'll be reading this advice having recently given birth, or even before, if you're well prepared. In which case you can implement the advice to rest, and introduce pelvic floor exercises into your routine as soon as you feel comfortable doing so. However, it's never too late to make improvements to your pelvic floor function, so don't worry that you've missed the window for recovery. Unfortunately, in the UK, you are not typically offered any physical postpartum assessment of your pelvis following birth unless you've had an obstetric tear of the anal sphincter injury, which is known to impact your pelvic floor and bowel function. In fact, your 6-week check-up with your doctor or OBGYN may not include any physical assessment at all. We would recommend that a pelvic floor assessment with a pelvic health physiotherapist/physical therapist is important for everyone after pregnancy. This is to identify how your pelvic floor is performing, and then you can begin a bespoke rehabilitation programme to ensure you are doing the exercises most suitable for you. This can help to prevent future problems and ensure you can return to exercise and the physical demands of motherhood safely. Many dysfunctions of the pelvic floor that can occur as a result of pregnancy and birth are not immediately obvious or symptomatic, but can present issues later on, so it's important to have it properly assessed.

What to expect during a pelvic floor assessment with a physiotherapist

A specialist physiotherapist will usually have the title 'Pelvic Health Physiotherapist' or 'Women's Health Physiotherapist' in the UK, and Pelvic Health Physical Therapist in the USA. They will have undergone post-graduate training and education to ensure they are qualified to carry out an internal assessment of your pelvic floor muscles and pelvic organs.

You'll spend some time with your therapist at the start of your appointment discussing your concerns or symptoms, and will be asked about your pregnancy/birth history, other gynaecological history and general medical history. Your therapist is likely to ask a few other questions and talk to you about your goals and fitness plans.

They will likely ask to look at your whole body, since many things can influence your pelvic floor function. This may include looking at your posture, asking you to perform a few simple movements and even watching how you breathe.

Your therapist should make you feel comfortable and explain the process of the internal assessment to you before you begin. You can ask them to slow down or stop at any time during the assessment. They will wear gloves and use lubrication to make the examination as comfortable as possible for you. They will insert one finger for the examination, so it is often much more comfortable than using a speculum, which you may have experienced in a smear test or other gynaecological exams. In most cases your pelvic exam will be performed in a lying position. You'll be asked to remove your underwear and be covered for your privacy. Sometimes it is beneficial to examine your pelvic floor in a standing position, particularly if this is when your symptoms occur, or for assessing your readiness to return to impact exercise. Again, you'll be assisted to cover yourself for privacy and your therapist should talk you through the assessment before starting, and ask your consent.

The aim of the pelvic exam is to feel how you are using the muscles and what actually happens when you do your pelvic floor exercises. Your therapist can also identify if there is any pain or discomfort when palpating the pelvic floor muscles, which might indicate some tension or tightness. The exam will also indicate the position of your pelvic organs, and be able to diagnose a prolapse. It is also possible to feel the tailbone (coccyx) and how it moves, which can sometimes be the source of pain after birth. This enables your therapist to then give you personal advice about what exercise you should be doing, things to avoid, and potentially identify areas that may benefit from treatment. This is often different for everyone, which is why physio-led pelvic floor exercises are recommended.

If any treatment is required, your therapist will explain this to you and create a treatment plan for you to consent to. This may include more hands-on therapy, exercise prescriptions or referral on to other services if necessary.

Questions to ask your pelvic health physiotherapist

- Do you specialize in pre-/postpartum health? (Not all pelvic health therapists will – there are many specialties within women's health.)
- Are you able to do an internal assessment of my pelvis and pelvic floor muscles?
- Can you assess and treat my C-section scar?
- Do you offer internal pelvic floor treatment?
- When would you recommend I book in for my postpartum assessment? (This is usually recommended around 6–8 weeks post-birth unless you need specific support for pain management or injury).
- After your assessment you may want to ask how many sessions they expect you to need if treatment is recommended.
- If you plan to cover the cost of your sessions with private medical insurance you need to check whether your therapist can accommodate this.
- Do you work with or have a local network of postpartum experts that you can connect me with? For example, doctors, fitness professionals, nutritionists, birth trauma counsellors, sexual therapists or psychologists. (This may not be necessary in your case, but it's good to know that your therapist can make personal recommendations if required.)

Never be afraid to ask your therapist to explain their findings, or what their clinical reasoning is behind the treatment plan they are recommending. It's important you understand what is happening with your body and what you can expect to achieve with treatment or an exercise plan.

How to find a qualified physiotherapist/physical therapist

Use the QR codes to direct you to the resources we've listed below.

POGP Directory

https://thepogp.co.uk/patients/physiotherapists (UK)

Mummy MOT Directory Link

https://www.themummymot.com/for-mums/
certified-mummy-mot-practitioners/

Squeezy App Directory for NHS and Private Pelvic Health Physio

https://squeezyapp.com/directory/ (UK)

Pelvic Global Directory

https://pelvicglobal.com/login/ (USA)

Pelvic Rehab

https://pelvicrehab.com/ (USA)

Academy of Pelvic Health Physical Therapy. Their website has a directory where you can locate a PT near you:

https://www.aptapelvichealth.org/ptlocator/

My birth story: Hazel

After a traumatic first (vaginal) birth with my son that left me with PTSD, I had a lot of anxiety around birth during my second pregnancy. I had experienced a severe haemorrhage and my son had been taken to intensive care while I was under general in theatre. I'd used hypnobirthing techniques during my pregnancy and labour, and all the things I had hoped for – skin-to-skin, immediate breastfeeding, a positive experience – went out the window and I was devastated. For various reasons, and following discussions with my consultant during my second pregnancy, I decided to have an elective C-section.

On the morning of my C-section I said goodbye to my son and my husband and I drove to the hospital – I felt really emotional at this point as I knew the next time I saw him we would be introducing him to his baby sibling (we didn't know we were having a girl). In theatre I had my amazing community midwife helping me to relax, my husband by my side, our playlist on the speakers and aromatherapy oils. The operating team were so calm and reassuring, and before I knew it my daughter was born, perfectly healthy. My husband was able to take photos and videos of the moment she was born. She was placed on my chest and we cuddled while I was stitched up and we took more photos. In the recovery room she was happy to start breastfeeding, and I enjoyed the classic hospital tea and toast.

I went home the following day, and my recovery was so much better than I expected. I had made a 'postnatal plan' while I was pregnant, so my husband and I both knew that we weren't going to have visitors for the first week or so, and my only 'job' was to feed my daughter and spend time with my son. By three weeks I was babywearing and at nine weeks I went for my first run, something I never would have thought would be possible so soon after a C-section. I think there is a lot of fear around C-sections, but my daughter's birth was such a positive experience and I would love to live the day all over again!

16

Incontinence issues after birth (and other toilet talk)

Leaking after birth can affect anyone, regardless of the type of delivery. Although statistics do suggest the risk for urinary incontinence is reduced as a result of a Caesarean birth versus a vaginal one,[8] many women will still experience incontinence symptoms in their lifetime, and having a C-section birth does not prevent this from happening.

Urinary incontinence or bowel incontinence (including passing wind) are common postpartum symptoms. Hang around a group of mothers and you'll probably hear someone making jokes about it. We want everyone to know that while it is common, it is not normal to continue to experience these problems beyond six weeks after birth. If you are still struggling with any leaking then you'll benefit from doing some pelvic floor therapy, and it's never too late to begin. Over 85 per cent of women who suffer with urinary incontinence resolve their issues by participating in physio-led pelvic floor therapy.[6, 9] The lack of open conversation about this topic due to embarrassment or fear is probably the reason that so many women don't know that help is available, or that this isn't simply an 'expected result of childbirth'.

There are different types of incontinence. Some are more widely discussed, while others may be less known. Women are more likely to experience some form of incontinence during pregnancy or after birth.

- **Urinary stress incontinence**: refers to leaking during activity or when there is an increase in pressure that affects the bladder – for example, when you run, jump, cough or sneeze. For some people this may be a very small amount, while for others it may be enough to need to wear pads regularly or interfere with their daily life.
- **Urge incontinence**: is caused by a sudden, frequent, intense urge to wee, which means you may not always be able to get to the toilet in time and leak as a result.

- **Overflow incontinence**: occurs when you can't fully empty your bladder when going to the toilet and may then experience some dribbling of urine that happens after.

It's possible to experience just one type of incontinence or a mixture of all of them.

These changes to your bladder function can occur for a number of reasons following pregnancy, including:

- Movement of the bladder or other pelvic organs, potentially resulting in a prolapse.
- Changes to the strength and function of the pelvic floor muscles, which help to control when the bladder neck and urethra opens and closes and the position of the bladder.
- Hormonal changes that occur during the third and fourth trimester, which can impact your bladder function and how the pelvic floor muscles behave.
- Adhesions from a C-section scar.

Often all these can be addressed with treatment successfully, but do require some assessment to ensure you are doing the right things, as no one rule fits all.

If you are struggling with urinary incontinence it's also worth considering how you can reduce irritation of the bladder with simple changes you can make at home. Irritants for the bladder include caffeine, alcohol, fizzy drinks and acidic or spicy foods. Try reducing or cutting these out of your routine for a while and see if you notice a change in your symptoms. Similarly, if you are in the habit of frequently trying to go for a wee 'just in case' then you're probably overstimulating the nerves, which send signals to the brain when the bladder is full and which can in turn lead to an 'overactive bladder'. If the bladder becomes used to storing less volume of urine before emptying, it can become harder for it to hold on as it fills. Retraining your bladder or changing these habits will take some time, but it is possible to do.

Similarly, bowel incontinence can occur following childbirth, with symptoms including increased urgency where you may struggle to get to the toilet in time, or the inability to control the muscles of the sphincter, which may result in staining in your underwear or soiling yourself. This can also occur when passing wind, as in some cases a person may lack the sensation to know the difference. Often these issues occur as a result of tearing of the sphincter muscles or nerves during a vaginal delivery. But in some cases this could still happen following a C-section birth if you've had a long labour first, with lots of pushing and straining to the rectum resulting in some nerve or muscle changes.

Constipation can also be a contributing factor to bowel incontinence, which can occur during pregnancy or following birth, so it is important to resolve this as soon as possible either with changes to your diet, increasing hydration or with medication.

Dealing with constipation after a C-section might be one of the things you're most scared about, and you're not alone! For so many, the thought of the first trip to the toilet causes a lot of anxiety – and unfortunately the more tense you are, the more uncomfortable it's likely to be. Try these simple tips to make the first stool easier to pass.

- Drink plenty of water – this will help to make the stool softer. Caffeine and alcohol are dehydrating so aim to avoid too much.
- Be mindful of your nutrition – avoid foods that usually don't agree with you and include lots of vegetables and fibre, which support good bowel habits.
- Use a small stool to put your feet on when going to the toilet, lifting your knees higher towards your hips. This helps to straighten out the rectum and relax the pelvic floor muscle which makes it easier to push out a bowel movement.
- Place a rolled towel or small cushion against your scar area and hold it in place with your hands as you go. This will make any pushing a little more comfortable.
- Try gently rocking back and forwards and slowly circling your hips if you're straining to go, this can also help to relax the pelvic floor muscles and reduce constant force or straining.
- Taking some deep breaths (similar to techniques you may have practised for birth) can be really helpful in reducing tension in the body and encouraging the pelvic floor muscles to relax.
- If necessary speak with your doctor about prescribing a laxative medication, because repetitive straining can cause pain, pelvic floor issues and haemorrhoids.

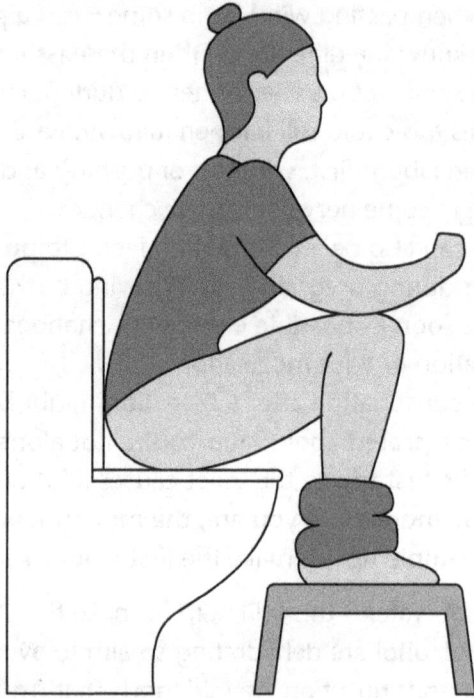

Figure 16.1 Using a small stool to put your feet on when going to the toilet helps to straighten out the rectum and relax the pelvic floor muscle which makes it easier to push out a bowel movement

Haemorrhoids (or piles) are enlarged blood vessels inside or around the anus and rectum. They are a common complaint during and after pregnancy as result of the increased pressure and force in the area. They can be extremely uncomfortable, cause bleeding, itching or protrude as a lump from the anus. They may affect your bowel habits, either due to pain and withholding, or in severe cases, because they may prevent the anus from closing completely, they can contribute to episodes of incontinence. Your doctor can prescribe treatment for piles, and certain changes to your lifestyle, toileting habits, diet, and pelvic floor therapy can all help too, so don't suffer in silence.

Gas after a C-section is common, and can be very painful. It can cause abdominal pain, pelvic pain and even severe shoulder pain. Bloating, gassiness and increased flatulence are all normal after a C-section, and can be caused by the effects of surgery, a slow digestive system and hormone changes occurring during the postpartum phase. Some things that may help to ease your discomfort are:

- Peppermint tea (we often get asked whether this will impact milk supply, but there is no scientific evidence of this and the NHS do not advise against drinking peppermint tea. Make your own informed decisions, but for many this can give real relief).
- Eat slowly – we know it's a rare treat to be able to sit down and take your time over a meal when you have a newborn, but sitting upright, chewing slowly and not rushing does really help to reduce painful wind.
- Be aware of foods that make it worse, and try to avoid them while you're still in the early days of recovery. This may vary from person to person but typically include gluten, highly processed food, dairy or carbonated soda drinks.
- Gentle movements and exercise such as some yoga poses, gentle stretching or short walks can help to get your digestive system working and reduce trapped gas.
- Heat pads or a hot water bottle may help to ease pain and discomfort.
- Don't be embarrassed to let the wind out! Honestly, the relief is worth it.

Other lifestyle factors that can contribute to incontinence include:

- Smoking
- Being overweight.

Hopefully, the more we normalize these conversations and spread awareness of all the management options we have for treating postpartum incontinence, the more we remove the taboo around it. Half of all women will experience urinary incontinence at some time in their lives, yet statistics show that over 30 per cent are too embarrassed to consult their doctor about their problem[10] and assume their bladder control will improve on its own.[11] Many women who experience daily symptoms of urinary incontinence do not seek help because they believe it is not abnormal.[12] If you're reading this and have been struggling with any of these symptoms, please know that help is available, and there is a very high success rate when you get the right treatment – and tell your friends, too!

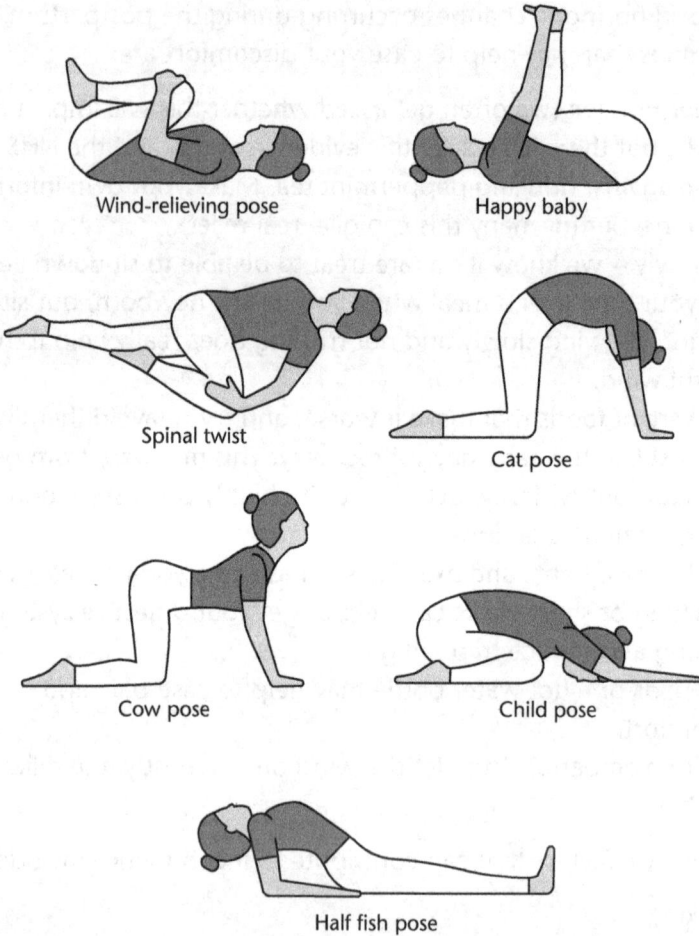

Figure 16.2 Gentle yoga poses can help with digestion and reduce trapped gas

Across the world there are different examples of postpartum care, which evidence the benefit of offering pelvic floor therapy post-birth. For example, in France women are offered ten sessions of physiotherapy after *every* birth, paid for by the state. Evidence tells us that increasing the level of education is an important factor in reducing the incidence of urinary incontinence in the elderly[13], so investing in pelvic floor therapy after birth could make a difference to your long-term wellbeing.

17

Prolapse

Pelvic organ prolapse (POP) is very common, affecting around one in three women who have had children. It can affect women after C-section birth or vaginal birth, and is usually the result of increased pressure and weight on the pelvic organs (bladder, bowel and uterus) and pelvic floor muscles during pregnancy, rather than the birth itself. Although a Caesarean delivery does reduce your risk of having a POP compared to a vaginal delivery, it does not completely remove the risk[8], so you should still be aware of the signs and symptoms. If you've had a previous pregnancy that resulted in a vaginal delivery, then this information may be even more relevant.

Our pelvic organs are supported by a group of muscles and ligaments called the pelvic floor, which also control the bladder and bowel function and help to prevent incontinence. They tolerate a lot during pregnancy, as the weight and downwards pressure increases as your bump grows, and they are affected by whichever type of delivery you've had, which is why we want everyone to feel confident about how to practise pelvic floor exercises after birth.

Many women describe their symptoms from a prolapse as being worse at certain times of day, or at certain times in their menstrual cycle. You may also notice specific activities will make your symptoms feel worse, such as opening your bowels, being on your feet for long periods of time or carrying heavy things. This is simply due to the effect of gravity, fatigue by the end of the day, or straining downwards. It's harder for the muscles to support the position of our organs if they have to also work against extra loads such as shopping bags or lifting and carrying a heavy baby.

A POP is defined as 'the downward movement of one or more of the walls of the vagina'. This may be the front (anterior) wall, back (posterior) wall or the uterus.

At least one pelvic organ (bladder, bowel, rectum or uterus) descends, causing a sensation of something 'pulling down' or a 'heaviness' or

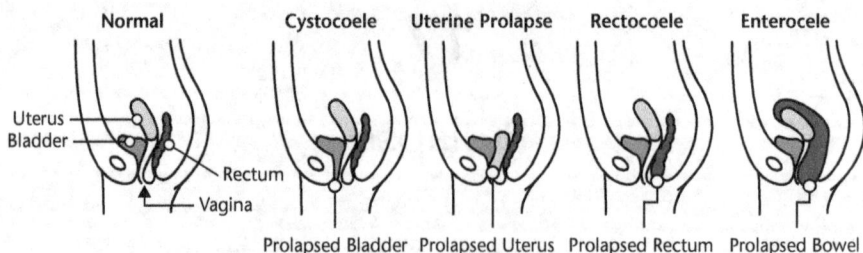

| Normal | Cystocoele | Uterine Prolapse | Rectocoele | Enterocele |

Uterus
Bladder
Rectum
Vagina

Prolapsed Bladder Prolapsed Uterus Prolapsed Rectum Prolapsed Bowel

Figure 17.1 different types of prolapse

'dragging' in the vagina. A bulge may be felt inside or outside of the vagina. Other associated symptoms may include lower abdominal pain, back pain, urinary or bowel leaking or a feeling of not being able to fully empty the bladder or bowel, constipation or pain during sex.

The extent of the movement can be assessed and graded by a medical professional such as a family doctor, nurse practitioner, OBGYN or pelvic health physiotherapist. In the UK, you will not typically be assessed for this at your postpartum check, but you can ask them to do an internal physical assessment if you have symptoms or concerns. The majority will be a low grade (Grade 1–2), and can be managed with conservative treatment such as physiotherapy, exercises, movement modification, toileting advice and good nutrition to support bladder and bowel function. There are also some products that help to support the position of the pelvic organ, support the function of the pelvic floor muscles or support the vaginal wall, such as a pessary.

More severely graded prolapses (Grade 3–4) may require surgical management. This usually applies when there has been a lot of movement or the descent of the vaginal wall or organ is felt at the vaginal entrance, or has moved externally. A consultant may also advise treatment if you are struggling with significant symptoms that affect your daily function or quality of life.

Other non-surgical options include using a pessary to support the prolapsed organ. This can be fitted by a specialist doctor, nurse or physiotherapist. A pessary is a medical device that can be inserted into the vagina to provide support to the vaginal wall that may have been displaced by the movement of a pelvic organ. There are many different shapes and sizes of pessary, and it may take a few attempts to find the right fit for you. When inserted correctly they should not be uncomfortable, and will usually be replaced every 3–6 months. You will be able to resume all of your normal activities, including sex, while it is in place. If you are concerned, make an appointment with your healthcare provider, doctor, or a pelvic health physiotherapist to get a proper assessment.

It is possible for a pelvic organ prolapse to improve after pregnancy and birth. Very mild prolapses may improve or even go away after a few months when your hormones return to normal levels, or as your pelvic floor muscles recover. However, this is not the case for everyone and it's more common for your prolapse to be managed with conservative treatment, rather than resolved. This is important, since a lower grade prolapse is unlikely to impact your daily life, so you'd want to maintain it at this level.

Physiotherapy-led pelvic floor exercises are proven to be effective in improving prolapse symptoms. Other simple changes that can make a big difference include diaphragmatic breathing, modified exercise, posture correction and education.

It is possible for a pelvic organ prolapse to get worse. The tissue is vulnerable to increased pressure or force, and also to hormonal changes. For this reason, some women will experience a worsening of symptoms around the menopause when the decline in levels of oestrogen impacts the pelvic floor muscle tone and function. Posture, activity and daily habits can all influence how much force or pressure you put on the pelvic floor and pelvic organs. For example:

- Regular straining on the toilet, episodes of constipation
- A repetitive cough
- Chronic vomiting (women who suffer with extreme morning sickness or hyperemesis during pregnancy may have a greater risk)
- Holding in a sneeze
- Holding or sucking in your tummy muscles for long periods
- Wearing tight waistbands/clothing around your middle for long periods
- Slumping or slouching while sitting so that your middle is compressed
- Heavy lifting – particularly overhead lifting, pushing, pulling
- Being overweight
- Returning to some forms of exercise too quickly after birth before the pelvic floor has recovered.

Many of these are things you can change or manage better if you know that a prolapse has occurred. Being fully informed means that you can make lifestyle and exercise choices that can help to prevent a prolapse from getting worse now or as you get older.

It can be easy to become fearful of movement or exercise when you are told you have a prolapse. It is important at first to modify exercise and to learn how to perform them correctly so that your pelvic floor and core is functioning properly. But maintaining a good level of strength and fitness is really important for prolapse management. The stronger your other muscles are, the more they will support the pelvic floor muscles during activity; this means there is less strain on them. Maintaining a healthy weight also reduces strain on the prolapse and pelvic floor. Because we know that during menopause women lose muscle mass and strength naturally, it's essential to regain as much strength and muscle as possible following pregnancy and postpartum, so that we have more 'in the bank' for when this time comes to avoid that decline in strength having a negative impact on a prolapse later on.

A prolapse diagnosis does not mean it will get worse if you choose to have another pregnancy. For many, the knowledge that they have a prolapse means they will be more mindful of how they look after their body during another pregnancy. If you've learnt strategies such as diaphragmatic breathing techniques, exercises to strengthen your core and pelvic floor, posture correction and know the things to avoid, your pelvic floor may cope better this time around. Having the confidence and information to approach your postpartum recovery differently can also impact how well you recover the next time. You should discuss your birth plan with your birth team as there are things you can do to prevent excess strain during birth, which reduces your risk of POP occurring if you choose to try for a vaginal delivery the next time. If you feel anxious, working with a pelvic health physiotherapist during your pregnancy can really help.

18

Managing birth trauma after your C-section experience

In our roles as a Physiotherapist and Scar Massage Therapist, our primary involvement with C-section recovery is the physical side. However, we really recognize that often it is impossible to achieve good physical outcomes if a mother is struggling mentally after birth. If you've read through the rest of this book, you'll know by now that tension in the body can impact pelvic floor function, core engagement, your breathing capacity and can be a contributing cause of pain. Often, a traumatic birth experience or postpartum anxiety or depression will result in more tension or higher pain levels. If you have negative associations with your birth this may be the reason you feel unable or uncomfortable to look at or touch your C-section scar.

Good postpartum recovery does rely on the mother being able to prioritize her own self-care, even if just for short periods of time, but often if you are struggling mentally it is unlikely you'll have the energy or motivation to commit to these self-care practices. In this case, you may need support to overcome these overwhelming emotions first, before your physical recovery can really progress. We believe in a holistic approach to care, combining physical recovery with good advice about rest, nutrition and addressing mental wellbeing when necessary. For this reason we've sought the expertise of Tracy Law, a Birth Trauma Counsellor and former midwife, to share her advice in this chapter.

Birth matters – it matters how you birthed, what you went through, and the surrounding events you encountered. Whether that's the impact the pregnancy or birthing experience had on your body, the way you were treated, how you were spoken to, or how you were made to feel. With birth being the doorway into parenthood, what we experience can colour our entire birthing and parenting experience, paving the way for either an exciting or fearful journey ahead.

Research evidence shows that 4-5% of women develop post-traumatic stress disorder (PTSD) every year after giving birth[14], amounting to approximately 30,000 women in the UK, while about a third of women experience birth as traumatic. It is often understood that traumatic experiences are situations posing a threat to life or safety, however this is not always the case. Trauma can be a result of any situation that leaves you feeling overwhelmed or isolated, even if it doesn't involve physical harm. In fact, it can be anything that felt too much, too soon or too quick for your nervous system and body. It can also be what didn't happen, what should've happened, or what could've happened in the absence of resources, care, connection and support needed at the time of your experience. Therefore, it is important to acknowledge the possibilities for trauma when it comes to the prenatal period, labour, and postnatal experience – birth trauma is real and valid, no matter how or why it came about.

Birth trauma can encompass a variety of experiences, including unexpected medical interventions, surgical procedures such as elective and emergency C-sections, and situations where you felt afraid, out of control or helpless. Long, difficult labours and short, intense ones can both be traumatic. Having a premature or ill baby who requires time in special care can be traumatic. A C-section, though often necessary for several reasons, can be traumatic. Each of these experiences, alongside many others, can have a profound effect on both your physical and mental wellbeing. At times, birth trauma even results in post-traumatic stress disorder. Subsequently, such events may not only affect how you feel during these moments in time, but they may also impact how you are able to live your day-to-day life following the event. Therefore, understanding the complexity of birth is important when accessing effective support for your healing journey, because that support is available, and healing is possible.

Throughout my time working as a midwife, perinatal practitioner, and now birth trauma practitioner, I have heard countless stories of birth trauma – each of which are completely unique and subjective to the individuals who experienced them. They vary from the detailed stories of harm caused to bodies during labour, to simple yet painful comments such as 'at least your baby is healthy', which inadvertently invalidate difficult birth experiences and worsen mental and physical health challenges. One example of these vastly differing experiences can be seen through the feedback I have received from clients who have birthed with a C-section – for some it can feel traumatic, and for others it can feel redemptive and healing. Feedback serves to highlight the varied experiences individuals have with C-sections. Each story differs, shedding light on the emotional complexities and challenges faced by those who have undergone this surgical birth method.

I hear stories of very long, difficult and painful labours that result in an emergency C-section, whilst others tell me of their elective Caesarean, chosen out of fear from previous traumatic births, for medical reasons, or due to complications during pregnancy. I hear of general anaesthesia and epidurals being cause for both calm and panicked births. Yet, despite the differing stories, one thing remains constant – most women want to know that they can be supported in their choices and given the help to recover. So, in understanding the physical and mental dimensions of a Caesarean section, it allows for a better understanding of the procedure's full impact and offers an opportunity to better navigate the potential complexities of this birthing experience.

However, this understanding and support may not have been your own experience. Maybe your birth left you feeling scared, overwhelmed, frustrated, ignored, sad or guilty, and has resulted in intrusive thoughts, flashbacks or nightmares related to the traumatic event. Maybe you find yourself constantly replaying the birth experience in your mind, leading you to avoid hospitals or pregnant friends, and struggle with sleep disturbances. This heightened state of alertness can also make you feel constantly on edge and perceive the world as unsafe, often profoundly impacting a mother's sense of self, parenting confidence and overall mental wellbeing. Common emotions such as guilt, shame and disappointment may often arise, particularly if the birth deviates from expectations, and these feelings can hinder bonding with the baby and the transition to motherhood. To address these impacts of birth trauma, acknowledging and validating emotions surrounding the event are the first steps needing to be taken in order to move forwards in your healing journey.

When stress and chronic pressures overwhelm the body, it responds intelligently, preparing to confront external threats. However, this response can become dysregulated, leading to states of hyper- or hypo-arousal and various forms of self-protection. What remains unprocessed may manifest in physical symptoms, as the body seeks ways to express suppressed worries or traumas. Exploring areas of the body commonly affected by emotional trauma, such as the jaw, diaphragm, pelvic floor and psoas muscle, is crucial in addressing these symptoms. These spaces within the body often hold unprocessed experiences, and acknowledging their significance is essential for understanding and treating chronic, unexplained symptoms.

When dealing with the implications of a Caesarean section, the psychological toll can be profound and multifaceted. For many of you, a Caesarean isn't just a procedure; it's a twist in your birthing plan, stirring up a mix of emotions that linger long into your postpartum period. It can be a moment where anticipation meets uncertainty, and the road to motherhood takes an unexpected turn. C-sections deviating from one's birth plan or expectations can evoke a sense of grief or uncertainty, impacting one's sense of self and parenting confidence. This may manifest as anxiety, depression and port-traumatic stress disorder (PTSD). For mothers who have undergone C-sections, the physical recovery process often intersects with the emotional impact of birth trauma – the C-section scar serves as a visible and tangible reminder of the childbirth experience, possibly evoking a range of emotions, from pride to distress. Physical discomfort, mobility limitations and body image concerns may contribute to the emotional toll of C-section recovery, especially for those who did not anticipate or plan for a surgical birth. Therefore, supportive postpartum care is vital for C-section recovery and healing from birth trauma. Practical assistance with tasks, childcare and self-care can alleviate stress, and allows individuals to prioritize emotional well-being. Additionally, open communication with healthcare providers, peer support, and professional services are crucial steps in the healing process. This is where birth trauma specialists can help.

Offering empathetic listening, validation and tailored coping strategies, birth trauma practitioners provide a non-judgmental space for exploring emotions, processing experiences, and developing coping mechanisms through therapy sessions and specialized techniques. Such sessions are the key to empowering and equipping mothers to manage symptoms, regain emotional control and access power over their experiences. By processing the traumatic memories surrounding certain events, trauma specialists are able to facilitate moving forward in the healing journey. It is through techniques such as stabilization and resourcing, trauma-informed debriefs, the rewind technique, and somatic and compassionate inquiry work, that individuals can revisit and reprocess traumatic experiences in a safe and controlled environment. This approach allows for the integration of past events, reducing their emotional intensity and enabling individuals to navigate their healing journey with greater resilience and clarity.

Understanding the signs and symptoms of trauma and PTSD is vital, and can help individuals find the necessary tools to move forward. PTSD is caused by the failure of the brain to process memories in the normal way, with these memories being stored in the wrong part of the brain. Consequently, this deviation leads to the past traumas feeling very real and present within current daily life. Symptoms may include intrusive thoughts or memories of the traumatic event, avoidance of reminders and heightened negative emotions or feelings of threat. Perhaps the event replays in your mind, over and over again, like a film loop? Everyone experiences PTSD differently, however almost all describe themselves to be struggling with loneliness, anxiety and exhaustion. In some cases, due to lack of awareness and education, these descriptions may have led to incorrect diagnoses by doctors, often being wrongly identified as postnatal depression. Whilst both illnesses share some symptoms, they are in fact entirely separate and require different treatments – PTSD symptoms can be treated quickly and often without medication.

When treating PTSD, it is important to recognize that this manifestation of trauma is a result of your brain's protective response to what it perceived was a threat. You may find yourself asking, 'what if...?' or 'if only...?' as you try to make sense of why your body has gone into a survival-based response – shutting down or freezing – and the memories feel overwhelming and unmanageable. Traumatic memories are often stored as sensory elements without words, comprising images, emotions and thoughts, which are often involuntarily recalled. This is due to the prefrontal cortex of your brain being offline during the traumatic event, making it difficult to process events logically and reasonably, and subsequently leading to memories resurfacing when we least expect them. These symptoms are your mind's attempt to make sense of an extremely scary situation. However, despite this being an involuntary response to trauma, with professional support and guidance it is possible to rewire how your brain cognitively processes these memories. Therefore, seeking support for stored traumatic experiences can gradually bring the system back into regulation, signalling to the body that the past is no longer present, and it is safe to emerge from the state of active self-protection you are in. This form of nervous system regulation is vital in addressing the impact of birth trauma, and plays a major role within my practice as a birth trauma specialist.

Therefore, by seeking specialist support to understand how the nervous system responds to stress and trauma, individuals can be empowered to develop effective coping strategies and promote their own healing. Education around nervous system regulation involves providing tools and techniques to help regulate physiological responses to stress and trauma, such as deep breathing exercises, progressive muscle relaxation, mindfulness practices and grounding techniques, aiding in calming the nervous system and reducing the intensity of emotional responses. Subsequently, through learning and putting into practice these specialized techniques, healing from birth trauma is an exciting reality for many looking to regain control over their experiences. Reaching out for help can be nerve-racking, but taking this first step might be the beginning of a life free from birth trauma – empowered, equipped and fully in control.

Useful resources

Use the QR codes to direct you to the resources we've listed below.

birthtraumaresolutionbrighton.com

birthtraumaassociation.org.uk

makebirthbetter.org

netmums.com

samaritans.org

miscarriageassociation.org.uk

birthrights.org.uk

sands.org.uk

Visit Your local GP surgery
Visit Accident and Emergency at your nearest hospital
Call NHS – 111
Samaritans – 116 123
CALM – 0800 58 58 58
Text SHOUT to 85258 to start a confidential conversation

My birth story: Lucy

My birth stories are far from textbook. When we discovered we were pregnant in December 2017, it was a shock to say the least. We booked an early scan because it didn't feel real until we saw that tiny, diamond ring shape on the screen – the flicker of life. This pregnancy seemed standard, or so I thought. I endured awful morning sickness and constant tiredness. But then, at our 20-week scan, the sonographers face dropped, and our dream turned dark.

I had a septate uterus, something no one had warned us about. Our daughter's head was stuck between the septum and my cervix. We were told she would likely need a tracheotomy at birth due to improper neck formation and would have life-long disabilities. She had talipes on both feet, visible in every scan. In hospital, we saw the casts she'd need from birth and the boots and bars she'd have to wear until she was five. For our first baby, this was overwhelming.

Then, at 28 weeks, I sensed something was wrong. At our local hospital I was blue-lighted to another specialist centre. We saw the plastic bag our baby girl would be placed in, too premature to hold heat. They pumped me full of magnesium and steroids to prepare her brain and lungs for the outside world. They halted contractions, but at 31 weeks, labour could not be stopped. I drove back to the local hospital, where they started the magnesium drip.

Frantic calls were made to find a NICU bed for our baby and a ward for me. The closest place was in London. The ambulance arrived, but they couldn't take my partner. He had to head home and find a train to London. I arrived at midnight, and after six hours of monitoring, the decision was made to do an emergency C-section. We had the head of NICU, ENT specialists, midwives, and an anesthetist – all in that small operating theatre, uncertain of our baby's condition. At 4:01 p.m., Grace was born, weighing 3 lb 9 oz. She wasn't breathing, had to be resuscitated, and was ventilated before being taken to intensive care. I didn't get to hold her. I didn't even get to see her. She was there, and then she was gone. They wouldn't let me see her until I could walk unaided, had my catheter removed, and had eaten without vomiting. I don't think they anticipated my reaction because, within two hours after my emergency C-section, I was up. Nothing could stop me. I don't remember the pain; I just remember feeling like my heart had been ripped out and placed in an incubator in NICU. I felt I had to be near her to breathe.

Grace stayed in the hospital for eight weeks, between London and our local hospital. Life as a NICU parent is like playing snakes and ladders, and nothing could be truer. Our remarkable little girl self-corrected on every issue she had. Her only battle scars are tiny marks on her feet from daily blood gas tests and an indent on her nose from being squashed inside me and then needing a breathing tube for eight weeks.

Then came our second miracle baby. After Grace was born, we knew we couldn't risk going through that again. Even if it was a one-in-a-million chance, it was too much. I had surgery in 2020 to remove the septum as much as possible to create a better chance for another baby, should we be so lucky.

We fell pregnant in December 2020. This pregnancy, though heavily monitored due to concerns about the placenta growing into scar tissue, went beautifully. I had the most amazing baby bump, something I never experienced with Grace. We had a scheduled C-section planned, but life had other plans. I went into labour a week early, after a particularly stressful day when Grace caught COVID. I drove myself to the hospital alone. Rosie, our second daughter, was breech, so I had another emergency C-section at 4:21 a.m. on August 12, 2021. It was just Rosie and me for 24 hours, and though it wasn't what we had hoped for, I held her skin-to-skin the entire time. I started our breastfeeding journey – just me and her. My beautiful 8 lb 9 oz baby girl pieced back together parts of my broken heart from my first birth with Grace.

Nothing about my story is what I thought pregnancy and birth would be. It was nothing like the books or movies. I've since had two miscarriages and am still learning just what a miracle pregnancy and birth are. How special a woman's body is – the strength it must show, the pain it endures and the love it holds. It is nothing short of remarkable.

19

Intercourse after a C-section

Most health professionals will recommend allowing 4–6 weeks of recovery before having sex after both a vaginal and a C-section birth, but it's very often an individual experience. It's also completely normal to wait much longer than that so you shouldn't feel any pressure to try until you feel ready. It is possible to get pregnant again as little as three weeks after delivery, even if you're breastfeeding. This is why contraception is discussed at your 6-week postpartum doctor's appointment.

You should be aware that it's normal to experience postpartum bleeding called lochia for up to six weeks after birth. This applies to C-section delivery too. It takes approximately six weeks for the uterus to return to normal size and for the cervix to close completely (even after a planned C-section birth when you haven't gone into labour, your cervix will open), and therefore the risk of infection is higher during that time. This is also likely to be around the same time that your C-section wound has fully closed. It can take longer for internal and external healing to happen if you suffered with any post-birth complications, and so we'd recommend seeking professional advice before resuming sexual activity.

Studies have reported 91.3 per cent of women will experience at least one sexual problem in the postpartum period[15], and yet it is rarely covered or discussed in pre-or postnatal appointments with a health professional. Often women will feel embarrassed or unable to ask these questions, but it is important to clarify that this should not be accepted as normal.

Many women will have moved through stages of labour before having a C-section that impacts their pelvic floor muscles. Even in the case of an elective C-section, the pelvic floor muscles are under significant strain for the duration of the pregnancy, which causes them to change and behave differently during postpartum. This may have an impact on your sex life, and women regularly report that intercourse feels different, uncomfortable or even painful after birth.

While many people assume that pregnancy and birth causes the pelvic floor to weaken or 'stretch', it's actually very common for the muscles to hold tension as a result of being under so much strain, or due to a birth experience that may have been difficult or traumatic. This sustained tension means the muscles don't move through a normal range of motion as easily, which can eventually cause pain or discomfort or be the cause of leaking. This is even more likely to occur when you are very tired, emotional or anxious as the body has a physical response (you might be more familiar with tension headaches, a clenched jaw or craving a massage – but it's a similar response local to the pelvic floor muscles).

Feeling anxious before intercourse can make pelvic floor muscles tighten up in anticipation of pain or discomfort, especially the first time. This in turn is likely to make it more uncomfortable to have penetrative sex and can become a bit of a vicious circle. Have open conversations with your partner, and let them know you may need to take things slower, spend more time on foreplay or try different positions to make you comfortable. You might choose to also include other things that usually help you to relax. Persistent pain during sex is called dyspareunia and is a treatable condition, so do seek help if things don't improve.

Pelvic floor exercises can encourage your muscles to fully relax as well as squeeze and engage, and this is really important because overly tight muscles can contribute to painful sex. Take a look at Chapter 15 to ensure you are performing your exercises correctly. Improving your pelvic floor function can also improve your sexual pleasure.

Breastfeeding and hormonal changes that cause a drop in oestrogen levels after birth can cause your vulva to feel drier than usual and the tissue can become thinner and more sensitive, so it is sensible to consider using lubrication to make it more comfortable for you. We recommend Yes! organic lube or natural products without synthetic chemicals. You can also apply vaginal moisturizers to help treat the area if you are noticing any sensitivity such as discomfort when wearing underwear or when sitting. Try to avoid using perfumed soaps or washes when you bathe as these often change the natural PH of your vagina and can cause further irritation.

A C-section scar can continue to be sensitive for a very long time after it appears to have healed externally, and could feel painful in certain positions, or when compressed many years after delivery. This might be due to the nerves around the scar and tummy being more sensitive, or due to adhesions or tension at the scar site that cause pulling or tightness in the surrounding muscles, including the pelvic floor muscles. For a step-by step guide about how to treat this yourself, go to Chapter 24 on C-section scar massage'.

Use the QR code below to direct you to our Tiktok page for more videos about scar massage for some suggestions on how to treat this area yourself at home, and some alternative positions to reduce strain on your scar region during intercourse.

www.tiktok.com/@the360mama

If you have been diagnosed with a prolapse after birth, or have concerns that you may have one, it may be reassuring to hear that there is no evidence to suggest that vaginal sex makes a prolapse any worse or cause any damage to your uterus, rectum or bladder. So any changes you make should be about your own comfort and enjoyment.

Regular anal intercourse may impact the muscle tone of the sphincter as anal penetration stretches the sphincter beyond its normal limits. This could contribute to worsening rectal prolapse. If you have specific concerns about this it is best to seek the advice of a professional such as a gynaecologist or a pelvic health physiotherapist, who can offer more individual recommendations based on an assessment.

Some women with a prolapse do experience anxiety around sex, and this can affect libido, self-esteem and body confidence. Alongside possible changes to the laxity of vaginal tissue, and pelvic floor muscles, these can all impact your enjoyment of sex. If you feel uncomfortable then it is worth exploring other positions, such as propping your hips up on a pillow, because some may suit you better than others. It's highly unlikely your partner will feel anything different if you have a mild prolapse.[16] If you are finding that your prolapse is physically limiting for your sex life, you should seek medical support, because it is not something you should expect to live with. Psychosexual counsellors can be really helpful for supporting individuals or couples who are struggling with their relationship, experiencing altered libido, fear, emotional issues or pain with sex after birth.

20

Starting exercise after a C-section

Exercising after birth can be a confusing topic. General advice tends to suggest avoiding exercise for six weeks, but then there is little advice available to explain what exercise you should return to, or why six weeks is the right time to start. Our best way of explaining this guidance is to consider that six weeks is the *average* amount of time for the initial repair phase to occur, meaning the acute tissue injury or damage has healed. This might look like your scar being fully closed, scabs falling away and the skin not looking red, hot or sore. However, this is not an indication of how the deeper layers of tissue are recovering, or whether your core or pelvic floor muscles are functioning well, or whether they need some rehabilitation. The average healing time does not necessarily apply to you, and so we recommend you really listen to how your body is feeling and if possible, seek a full body assessment with a specialist physiotherapist who can create a programme that is bespoke for you.

Vague guidelines that recommend returning to exercise at six weeks don't take into account what your fitness levels were like before birth, what birth experience you had, whether you had any complications in your recovery, or what type of exercise you might be planning to do. Therefore, it's not really very helpful. Hopefully most people do interpret that advice as a gradual return to exercise, but often, motivated to lose weight or to regain fitness, women will begin challenging fitness regimes at six weeks thinking they have given their bodies adequate time to heal.

Even after an uncomplicated pregnancy and birth, the body changes significantly and will require some rehabilitation to restore good function and form with exercise. This is a key time during which people may begin to move or perform exercises with compensations that will eventually lead to injury if not addressed. We recommend that all mothers complete a phase of reconnecting and strengthening with some specific targeted exercises to ensure they are addressing the changes in their body before going straight back to pre-pregnancy exercise or starting any new fitness routines or classes.

When planning a return to exercise you should also take into account how deconditioned your muscles are as a result of pregnancy, as many people stop exercising for a period of time either due to pregnancy aches and pains, tiredness or other medical reasons. For example, a mother who has continued to exercise regularly throughout her pregnancy would likely have a different return to exercise compared to someone who hasn't exercised for several months and is starting from a lower baseline of fitness and strength. This is no different from anyone else starting a new gym programme – an effective and safe programme would be developed based on your starting fitness levels.

Similarly, the suggestion that you'll be doing zero exercise at all for the first six weeks is also misleading. Most people will be starting to return to regular activities of daily living after a couple of weeks, and of course lifting and carrying a baby frequently. Even walking with a pram, lifting a car seat or bags of shopping requires some muscle activation and strength, so we shouldn't be fearful of doing some simple exercises that are less strenuous, as they can help to support the recovery of our core and pelvic floor muscles.

At the right time and at the right level, movement can really support your overall recovery, so to remove the fear associated with returning to exercise and provide you with a sensible plan of action, we've created a timeline to help guide you to know what to do and when. Please be aware that this is not a bespoke programme, and your recovery will be unique to your situation and you should always listen to your body. We'd advise having a postpartum assessment with a specialist physio-therapist to make a personal plan for your return to exercise.

An example of a safe return to exercise after a C-section:

PP Stage	Type of Exercise	What to avoid
0–2 weeks	Deep diaphragmatic breathing Pelvic floor exercises Walking little but often	Sitting up directly from lying or from a deep sofa. Instead roll onto your side and push up this way to avoid straining the core muscles or your scar. Lifting or carrying anything more than the weight of your baby and especially avoiding lifting anything overhead. Any movement that is painful to perform.

2–6 weeks	Pelvic floor exercises Deep core connection exercises in various positions Gentle stretching Posture correction Walking distance can gradually increase as you feel comfortable	Skipping the early steps of re-engaging with your deep core and pelvic floor muscles. Doing too much. Lochia is postpartum bleeding, which is expected to continue for up to six weeks. Heavier bleeding, pain or general malaise is a sign you're pushing yourself too much.
6–12 weeks	Pelvic floor exercises Progress core exercises with more load or challenge Functional strengthening such as squats / lunges Stretching Gentle yoga Gentle Pilates Avoid heavy impact exercise	Skipping the strengthening stage and adding in too much impact exercise too quickly. Even if you feel great after birth, your body has changed significantly throughout your pregnancy and birth. You'll benefit from getting stronger again before you start impact, HIIT or heavy resistance training.
12+ weeks	Return to impact exercise Gradual return to running Increasing load / resistance training Pilates Yoga	Not progressing the challenge level in your workouts. If you've moved through the steps above, your workout will need to progress now if you want to see change.

Over the next few chapters we'll introduce you to some examples of exercises you can begin at home to begin your recovery. We are unable to offer direct advice about how or when to return to specific sports because it will vary according to the individual, but we do strongly recommend seeking a full postpartum body assessment with a specialist physiotherapist.

My birth story: Megan

First birth

Trigger warning: traumatic birth and NICU stay

I had a Category 1 (the most emergency kind) C-section in 2021. I had been planning a home birth, but after days in on-and-off labour and my waters broken for more than 24 hours I went to hospital for an induction. I had been slowly dilating and was 4 cm when I arrived. The midwives continued to be positive and I was very keen for a vaginal delivery. After hours of ongoing labour I decided to have an epidural. This was something I hadn't wanted but was really quick and such an amazing relief after being in so much pain. I continued to labour for several more hours but I had stopped dilating, there was meconium (poo) in my waters and the baby became very distressed, and the decision was made for a C-section.

At this point I could hear the baby's heart rate was very fast and lots of people rushed into the room. I felt very unwell and shaky, and it turned out I had sepsis from an infection in my womb. I was very tired and my memory of events is hazy. It was discovered at this point that the baby was coming out face first and back-to-back and had become stuck (obstructed labour).

It was all very scary, and when I got to the theatre my epidural had worn off and I still had sensation just before they started the operation. I was suddenly then numb and it was then a very fast birth – minutes after starting the operation our baby was born. She was lifted up over the curtains, screaming, and we found out we had a daughter. The surgery went well with no complications for myself and we then had delayed cord clamping. We were planning with the medical team for my partner to hold the baby as I felt so unwell. However, when our daughter was examined by the doctors they realized she was very unwell, and not able to maintain her blood oxygen levels so she needed to be taken immediately to the neonatal intensive care unit.

We were in total shock and I was quite delirious. We were then lying in recovery crying without our baby. We were told she may not survive the night and she had been born with low blood oxygen levels and might have a brain injury and that only time would tell. I couldn't see her for ten hours until we were both stable. When she was ready I was wheeled up to the intensive care unit and saw her from my bed. I was in bed for 24 hours with a catheter and on strong antibiotics, and I slept solidly for almost 12 hours (which was a shock after waking up to wee all night while pregnant). I had always been terrified of having a catheter, but in the end it was such a relief and I didn't want it taken out. When I first got out of bed it was absolute agony, and I was given more strong painkillers. In the days after I also had developed an ileus (where your bowel freezes and stops working) and was vomiting and unable to poo.

Thankfully, the baby quickly stabilized and then I set about recovering and started to breastfeed. It was very challenging pumping while hooked up to lots of intravenous medications and not able to eat due to bowel complications, but with the support of the staff it worked out. I was first able to hold and breastfeed my baby after five days, and very luckily it felt completely instinctive and she latched immediately. I then had a totally exhausting 24 hours going up and down to breastfeed on NICU on demand. My legs swelled and I was in agony. I reached breaking point and took a break from direct feeding. The NICU staff apologized and said that they hadn't realized how ill I was and that I could have been having more of my medications brought to the NICU so I didn't have to go back and forth so much. It was also during the Covid pandemic during the birth, and I found the added stress of being often separated from my partner and not seeing my family for my whole time in hospital very overwhelming. When the baby came to the ward I was on my own with her for almost 24 hours, and found this very hard emotionally and physically.

We were both discharged from hospital after one week, and started a long recovery from the traumatic birth experience, C-section and a significant diastasis. I had always been very fit and healthy and had an image that I would bounce back from birth and be back running in no time. Walking felt very strange and I felt totally out of alignment and was tripping over regularly. I needed to take over-the-counter painkillers for eight weeks and felt absolutely shattered. I managed to exclusively breastfeed with the help of my partner, who would take the baby overnight and only wake me when she absolutely had to feed. Thankfully the baby thrived and became a happy vibrant child with no lasting injury from the birth. I struggled with PTSD from the birth experience and NICU stay and had counselling.

Overall now I feel very grateful for the fact that the C-section saved mine and my daughter's lives. Physically, my recovery took a lot longer than I expected before having a baby. The wound healed well and after some time I did some at-home massage. The scar was slightly numb but I had no lasting pain. I struggled with a very significant diastasis and was under hospital physio. I took my recovery very gradually, with postnatal-specific exercise classes and regular women's health physio. Shortly after a year, I could do a full Pilates class and started running. I achieved the fastest woman in my age category time at Parkrun about a year and a half after the birth, and felt particularly proud. After a long and patient recovery and lots of focus on core and pelvic floor work, exercise felt different and I always had to think more consciously about my core, but I was in some ways the strongest I had ever been.

Second birth

Following my first traumatic birth I knew that if I had another baby I would choose to have a Caesarean. Being able to choose a Caesarean actually played a huge part in me being able to go through with another pregnancy. I couldn't bear the thought of the unpredictability of going through labour again, and after having a baby in NICU from birth complications I needed to know I was choosing the birth with the least risks to the baby. The medical team were all very supportive of this, and I was booked for an elective C-section. I remember in the lead up to the birth I was very nervous.

Following a complicated first birth I was absolutely terrified something would go wrong, and even told my partner the night before the birth that I was worried I might die. In the lead up to the birth I was constantly annoyed by people who kept telling me the booked C-section was going to be a lovely, healing experience following my first birth. I just kept thinking, 'nobody tells someone going for any other kind of major abdominal surgery that it is going to be lovely'.

The staff at the hospital were aware I was anxious, and did everything they could to support me through the experience. On the day of the surgery I had a very supportive obstetrician and anaesthetist who kept me updated about the timings and kept asking if I had any requests. The atmosphere in the theatre was very calm. The birth felt quite slow, and from starting it took ten to 20 minutes till our baby was born. I had a bad headache from the spinal and felt dizzy, but the anaesthetist constantly talked to me and gave me medications to keep me comfortable. We found out we had a baby boy (despite a funny confusion when the umbilical cord was covering his penis) and he was lifted up screaming and looking exactly like our daughter, and I felt an instant rush of love for him. We did delayed cord clamping and he was then examined briefly. He then lay on my chest and we did skin-to-skin. He breastfed in the theatre whilst the operation was finished. We stayed skin-to-skin for a long time, then my partner held him and my mum came into recovery to meet him. I did feel amazed by how calm, safe and predominantly pain-free the birth had been, and I feel very grateful for modern medicine.

This time was very different from my first experience. I had the catheter out and was up and walking to the toilet after about eight hours. I was in pain but it was manageable. I was also much less tired than after my first birth where I was in labour for days and developed an infection. This time I planned to move as little as possible in the early days and really focus on my recovery. My partner stayed with me and the baby in hospital and this was a huge support. I was able to be discharged after one night (partly my choice). Compared to the first emergency C-section I had an organized house ready for recovering from a C-section with everything at the right height and within reach. The second and third days were very painful, especially when moving in bed, but the pain quickly improved. I found the pain much worse after too much movement. I tried to walk up the road after about one week but found I was in lots of pain and turned back and lay down. My old self would have definitely pushed on, but I was trying really hard to embrace resting and listening to my body.

I was very careful with my diet and drank plenty of water, and having had terrible issues with bowel complications and constipation the first time around I was very happy with normal poos this time around.

With my second baby I was really worried about not being able to lift my toddler (just over two years old) after the C-section. However, despite being so young she was amazing, and really accepted that I needed to recover, and didn't seem upset that I couldn't lift her. I bought her some stools so she could reach things herself and she actually seemed very happy she could help mummy and do more things independently. I also got as much help as possible from family and did manage to not lift my toddler for 6–8 weeks after the birth. The thing I actually strangely enjoyed still doing was cooking, as I found this was all at the right level without bending and twisting and I felt I could really focus on my nutrition.

Second time around I had a lot less pain but also found as time went on my scar was more numb and I had more of an overhang. I arranged to have some C-section massages, which really helped and also was really good for connecting back to the scar area positively. I found an understanding women's health physio and followed Pilates approaches, and started practising the core breath from my first postnatal recovery and during the pregnancy. I started 360 breathwork early and I instantly felt I had better control of my core, posture and balance than after my first C-section. I took the same approach as after my first C-section and gradually built up with postnatal exercise classes and women's health physio. My recovery is still ongoing, but overall my second C-section was unexpectedly calm and positive, and it was a healing experience.

21

Movement that can support your healing in the early days

Movement can be a really helpful tool to aid healing and speed up recovery when used in the correct way.

It can be easy to misinterpret this advice, and so we want to make it clear – small, gentle movements, little and often throughout the day is your goal. This might look like some bed stretches or a walk to and from the bathroom, or to make a cup of tea at frequent intervals, at most a short walk outside to get some fresh air – but only if it's not painful. This will help to prevent post-surgery complications such as blood clots, swelling, or sores. It can also be helpful to ease painful wind or constipation which are common after abdominal surgery. It does NOT mean you should be embarking on an exercise routine, pushing the buggy for hours round the park or doing lots of strenuous housework a few days after you return home.

Reframing how you think about exercise might help in this phase of your recovery. The reason for exercising at this stage is to support your body as it heals. You'll really benefit from doing deep breathing, pelvic floor exercises or gentle core engagement exercises in bed or on the floor. Anything that is expending energy that you don't have or causing you pain is not useful and may slow down your recovery.

Remember that on top of the physical impact of pregnancy, potentially labour, and surgery, you will also most likely be affected by lack of sleep. It requires a huge amount of energy for your body to repair itself, which will add to your levels of fatigue at this time. If you are using up your energy stores doing other things, it will make a difference to how well or how quickly your body heals. While we understand that this is not always easy to do, we strongly recommend that you plan to expend as little energy as possible in the first couple of weeks, and instead allow your body to use those resources to heal.

Another way to measure whether you are doing too much is to pay attention to the amount of postpartum bleeding you are experiencing.

It is normal to experience some bleeding (lochia) in the first six weeks after birth, but you should expect this to gradually reduce as the weeks pass. If you notice a change, in particular if the bleeding suddenly becomes heavier, this can be a sign that you're overdoing it. If you are still bleeding beyond six weeks, this can similarly be a sign that your body is taking longer to heal, but you should seek a medical opinion in this scenario too.

Here we've put together some examples of simple movements and exercises that you could be doing in the first few weeks after birth, as long as you feel safe to do so and are not experiencing any post-surgical complications. If you feel concerned you can also ask your midwife or healthcare provider for their advice about when to begin.

Diaphragmatic breathing

The diaphragm movement will directly influence your pelvic floor muscles as they work together in a system which behaves like a piston. As the diaphragm moves downwards during the inhale, the pelvic

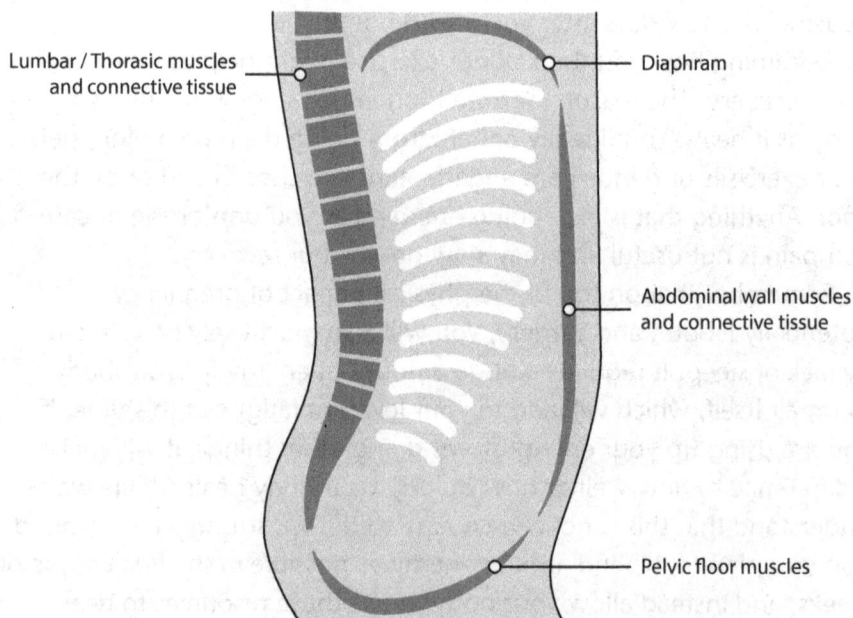

Figure 21.1 The diaphragm/pelvic floor piston

floor muscles move in the same direction, lengthening and relaxing to accommodate the increasing air pressure in our abdomen. As the diaphragm lifts upwards to push air out of our lungs during the exhale, the pressure in the abdominal region reduces and the pelvic floor muscles also lift upwards.

Therefore, even if you don't feel ready to begin pelvic floor exercises straight away, you can aid their recovery, and positively impact the core by introducing some breathing exercises that feel comfortable to do. This can help to reduce stress or anxiety and can easily be performed while you rest, feed or cuddle up with your baby.

You may have already read our instructions on diaphragmatic breathing earlier in the book, but if you're reading this chapter in isolation please find the information again here. To successfully perform a diaphragmatic breath, you should breathe in deeply through your nose. The lowest ribs should lift outwards, like two bucket handles lifting, as well as opening at the front and back. Your tummy should expand too. You could rest your hands lightly on the rib cage or tummy and feel for this movement as you breathe in.

Video: Diaphragmatic Breathing Tutorial #1

To follow video instructions of the exercises that follow in this chapter please use the QR code to visit our physio-led exercise library.

Exhale through your mouth, pursing your lips slightly. Make sure you fully complete the exhale, so there should be no breath left by the time you finish. If your hands are still resting on your rib cage you should feel them drop and move down and inwards as you complete the exhale. Your chest and tummy will also flatten.

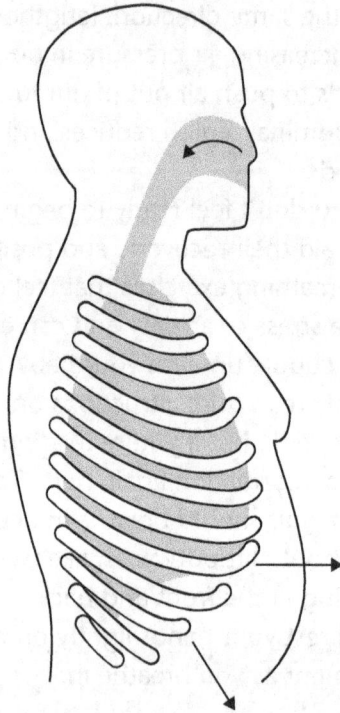

Figure 21.2 Diaphragmatic breathing

Start by just doing a few deep breaths at intervals throughout the day. You may find it easiest to practise them in a lying position at first, but when you become more familiar with them you can do them in any position.

This is a great starting point for eventually progressing to do more strengthening exercises for your core and pelvic floor. If you're reading this before giving birth, it is also something you can practise while pregnant and will mean you feel really familiar with the technique to begin again after birth as soon as possible.

For your C-section scar, this breathing technique also helps with early scar mobility, helping to prevent adhesions, tension or pulling from the scar later on. As your tummy gently rises and falls with the breath cycle, so does the scar tissue. This encourages better movement between the layers, improves blood flow to support healing and softly stimulates the nerve endings as they move, which can help to prevent pain, numbness, itching or altered sensation. Gradually you could

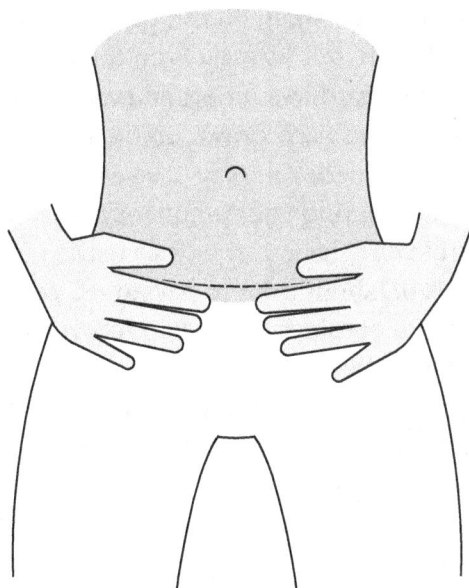

Figure 21.3 When exercising, if you touch your scar make sure your hands are clean or place them over a thin item of clothing

add light touch to the movement by laying your fingertips lightly over your scar and feeling the rise and fall of the lower abdomen. Bringing your awareness to the area, and gaining confidence in touching and interacting with your scar can be an important step to overcoming birth trauma, or negative emotions surrounding your scar. While it is not appropriate to begin scar massage for around eight weeks, this technique can be performed much earlier and introduces some of the benefits of massage from day one. Make sure if you're touching your scar directly your hands are clean or place your hands on your scar over a thin item of clothing.

Pelvic floor exercises

Pelvic floor rehabilitation can begin from day one after birth if you are comfortable to do so, but even before exercise one of the most beneficial things you can do for pelvic floor recovery is to rest. Taking weight or force off the pelvic floor muscles in the days after birth gives the muscles an opportunity to properly rest and recover.

Try to remember that the strain on this group of muscles comes not just from labour and birth, but actually from the pregnancy itself. The muscles work extremely hard to support an ever increasing weight and pressure as your bump and baby grows, so by the time you give birth they are usually very fatigued. You may have already experienced some pelvic floor dysfunction during your pregnancy, such as leaking urine, struggling to control wind, haemorrhoids or pelvic pain. If you have gone through stages of labour prior to having a C-section, you must also take this effort into consideration when recovering as this impacts the pelvic floor significantly too.

By allowing them a period of rest, (lying down is best as it completely offloads any downwards force to the pelvic floor), they have the opportunity to really recover, which means they are more likely to be able to work as required when you start doing more activity. In the same way that you might put your feet up for a few days after running a marathon – allow your pelvic floor muscles to do the same. When we are upright, our body weight, as well as the force of gravity, acts as a weight on top of the pelvic floor muscles. Any additional strain, such as carrying your baby, the buggy or car seat or a bag of shopping is all extra force on top of the muscles when they are vulnerable and tired. This can put you at greater risk of injury or dysfunction. Lots of women will describe feeling heaviness down below, or worry that everything 'feels like it's falling out' after giving birth. A few days spent resting can make a huge difference to how long those symptoms continue for.

Begin to exercise the pelvic floor muscles in offloaded positions for the same reason – it's easier for them to work when they aren't under strain. This might be lying on your back, or resting in child's pose.

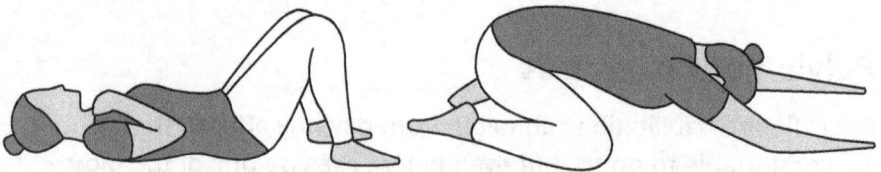

Figure 21.4 Exercise your pelvic floor in off-loaded positions such as lying on your back or child's pose

Breathe in deeply to relax the pelvic floor muscles; imagine you're sitting bones moving apart or melting into the floor. Breathe out through pursed lips as you lift the pelvic floor muscles into a squeeze. Aim to start from the back passage and lift up and forwards towards the front passage.

Visualizations can be helpful for some people. Here are some of the ones we use successfully with clients in our clinic:

- Lift from the back passage as if to stop yourself from passing wind, then lift and close your front passage as if to stop the flow of urine.
- Pull a zip closed starting from the tailbone and finishing at the pubic bone at the front.
- Imagine an elevator beginning in the basement and travelling up to the penthouse.
- Imagine drawing a tampon into your vagina to lift it up and away from the entrance.
- Imagine sucking a thick milkshake upwards through a straw.

Whatever works for you, you must also remember to release the effort and relax the muscles effectively between squeezes. Without this vital part of the exercise it is not possible to strengthen the muscles through their full range, meaning they can still struggle to perform properly in real life. Don't do pelvic floor exercises when going to the toilet as it can increase the risk of getting a urinary tract infection.

Using your breath in this way will ensure you are working slowly, and sustaining the squeeze as you complete a full exhale will work the control and endurance of the muscles, which is essential for good muscle function.

You will also need to practise faster repetitions, to mimic situations such as sneezing, coughing or jumping. In this scenario you should practise squeezing and releasing the muscles at a quicker rate; imagine your car indicator light blinking, and don't synchronize it with your breath. It should be easier to achieve this once you've improved your connection and confidence, and can isolate your effort to the local muscles.

Video: Recovery Exercises Tutorial #1

To follow video instructions of the exercises that follow in this chapter, please use the QR code to visit our physio-led exercise library.

'Bed Exercises'

Bed exercises

Early movement in bed is recommended to improve blood flow, circulation to prevent clots and flush away waste products and swelling, and to relieve stiffness, aches and pains. Your scar will also benefit from gentle movement and it can help to reduce adhesions, tugging or restriction when you do start moving around more in day-to-day life.

You can do these as soon as your pain is under control and you are stable after surgery. Some simple suggestions for you to practise in bed are:

Heel slides

Lie flat on your back with your legs extended. Breathe out as you slide one heel up the bed to bend the knee towards you. Inhale as you slide the heel slowly away to straighten the leg. Repeat on both sides.

Single knee drop

Lie flat on your back with both knees bent and the soles of your feet on the bed. Breathe in as you drop one knee out to the side until you feel a gentle stretch or pull across your tummy. Breathe out as you draw the knee back into the starting position. You should not move into a painful range, so at first it may be a small movement. Repeat on both sides.

Knee rolls

Lie flat on your back with your knees bent and keep your knees and ankles together. Slowly rock the knees over to one side until you feel a gentle stretch or pull across your tummy. Breathe out as you draw the knees back to the centre. Repeat in both directions.

Pelvic tilts

Lie flat on your back with your knees bent. Breathe out as you tip the pelvis backwards as if flattening your lower back into the mattress, then breathe in as you tilt the pelvis away from you to arch the lower back from the mattress. Repeat a few times within a comfortable range.

There are no set number of repetitions, instead listen to your body and move within a comfortable range. Little and often is likely to be better than doing one long session per day.

Video: Recovery Exercises Tutorial #2
'Chair Exercises'

Chair exercises

It's likely you'll spend a lot more time sitting at first, while you rest, feed or bond with your baby. This is a special time, but can leave you feeling a bit stiff, achy or noticing some pain in your neck, shoulders, back or hips. Introducing some easy exercises like these can help combat that, while also providing your scar with the opportunity to get used to some movements in a controlled way so that everyday movements are less likely to be painful or uncomfortable.

These exercises are likely to be appropriate for when you've returned home and you're feeling well enough to be moving around the house.

Thoracic rotations

Sit upright in a chair. Cross your arms over your chest and turn your torso to look over one shoulder. Return to the centre and repeat in the other direction.

Side stretch

Sit upright in a chair. Let your arms hang down beside you. Slowly lean over to slide one hand towards the floor and breathe in to feel a stretch. Breathe out as you lift yourself back to a seated position and repeat on the other side.

Pelvic tilts

The same movement you've performed on the bed. Breathe out to rock the pelvis backwards, imagine you're tucking your tail under. Breathe in to rock the pelvis the other way, arching your back and lifting your tail out behind you.

Single knee extension

Sit upright in a chair. Breathe out to straighten your knee and pull your toes back towards you, feeling your thigh muscles work. You may also feel a little bit of effort in your lower abdomen. Breathe in to lower.

Pumping ankles

It's common to get swelling post-surgery, and when we spend more time sitting down this can pool around your ankles and feet. To help reduce this swelling, try pumping your ankles by flexing and pointing the toes if they are up on a cushion, or marching your ankles on the spot on the floor at regular intervals to encourage better circulation.

Video: Recovery Exercises Tutorial #3

To follow video instructions of the exercises that follow in this chapter, please use the QR code to visit our physio-led exercise library.

'Standing Exercises'

Standing exercises

As you start to feel able, and you are becoming more active, you can progress to do some simple exercises in standing. This is really useful because they are more likely to mimic functional movement that you perform throughout the day and help to prepare your body for more activity.

These exercises are appropriate when you are feeling well, your pain is well managed and you might be starting to do more household chores, getting out for a short walk or feeling the urge to be more active.

Heel raises

Hold onto the back of a chair or surface. Lift up onto your tiptoes then lower back down, repeat a few times. This also helps to prevent swelling around your calves, ankles and feet.

Marching on the spot

Lift your knee towards your chest and lower, repeating from side to side. The higher you lift your knee the more you will be using your deep core muscles. This is a great way to start strengthening your core and reducing the lower tummy pooch often caused by a lack of connection or engagement with the lower tummy muscles after pregnancy and birth.

Side stretch

Stand tall with your hands resting by your thighs. Slowly lean to the side to slide one hand down the outside of your leg towards your knee. Take a deep breath in to increase the stretch, then exhale to straighten back up to standing. Repeat to the other side.

Overhead reach

You may feel some restriction with this movement at first as it can cause a pull to your scar. One of the outcomes of this is that people will compensate or move in a different way, eventually causing other postural or injury issues. You'll probably need to reach above you frequently throughout the day just to perform tasks around the house, so it's worth practising this in a controlled exercise so it doesn't take you by surprise.

Lean your back against a wall, move your feet a little away from the wall. Feel the back of your rib cage press against the surface. Raise one arm first with a straight elbow and wrist in front of you and then upwards towards the wall. Stop and notice where you feel restricted and then lower in the same arc back to your side. Do the same on the other side. Progress with one arm until you notice your range of motion increasing and, when you are comfortable, progress to doing the same movement with both arms at the same time. It may take several days or weeks to regain your full range of motion; be careful not to push through pain but just move to the edge of your restriction.

Hip circles

This will encourage some movement of your scar, as well as relieve stiffness in your hips and lower back.

Stand and hold onto the back of a chair or a surface. Lift one foot off the floor, bringing your knee towards your chest, and circle the hip around the socket in one direction, repeat a few times and then repeat in the other direction. Depending on your scar, you may start with small circles and build up to wider movement as your pain allows. It's OK to feel a bit of pulling, but it shouldn't cause pain. Repeat on both legs.

Roll downs

Stand with your back resting against the wall with your feet a little wider than your hips. Peel your spine slowly away from the wall, dropping your chin onto your chest and sliding your hands down your legs as far as you feel comfortable. Take a deep breath in to hold and then as you breathe out stack the spine back against the wall, standing tall.

Exercise as you recover should never be painful, and you should not feel exhausted after doing them. Listen to your body and stop if anything feels uncomfortable.

My birth story: Olivia

I was two weeks overdue and I was booked in for an induction. Three rounds of induction, 36 hours later, and still no developments. I'd heard of induction gels working fast when your body is close anyway, but clearly my baby wasn't budging anytime soon! The whole time I was being monitored and looked after, so I tried to stay calm and hoped that he would eventually make an appearance.

At the end of the second day I was offered a Caesarean, and I chose not to have it at that point – I hadn't had a single contraction at that stage and didn't feel like it was a necessary option. It wasn't the waterbirth I'd planned for and I wanted to try for that first. Fast-forward another 36 hours and I'd started having contractions that were three minutes apart, but doing nothing. Clearly the induction hormones had 'kicked in' all at once, but to no effect. I wasn't even 2 cm dilated, and they were unable to break my waters because I wasn't far enough along. By this stage (this was our fourth day in the hospital) I was exhausted, I'd barely slept, and they were worried about the baby's stress levels. I'd tried the tens machine and gas and air, and I thought I was managing it quite well, but it was difficult to manage the emotional roller-coaster when I had no idea how much longer this was going to take.

They eventually managed to break my waters and I was given an epidural. I went from 2–4 cm within an hour (whilst I slept) and I thought 'Great! This is it!' and then that ground to a halt and I was stuck at 4 cm for over four hours. Fortunately I wasn't in any pain, but they had found meconium in my waters and thought that it would be best to have a C-section for the safety of the baby. Although I had previously been a little apprehensive about having a C-section, once we'd made the decision I was impressed by how smoothly (and calmly) everything went. Immediately my partner was sent to change into scrubs and I was wheeled into surgery. In less than ten minutes the baby was pulled out, his cord was cut, and he was placed on my chest. Phew! To finally have him in my arms was such a relief after that long wait!

The surgical team and anaesthetist were all amazing. They didn't let on how concerned they were, and during the procedure they were surprisingly controlled and composed... I wouldn't go so far as to say it was peaceful because they were very busy, but it was nothing like I had imagined it to be. They absolutely filled me with confidence. I was wheeled into post-surgery and allowed to have hours of skin-to-skin and to try and initiate feeding. I'd feared that the recovery would be very slow and painful.

I'll admit the first two nights were difficult and it was strange not to be able to rely on my core muscles to move around in bed. However, on day three I was feeling well enough to go home and walk around the house and pick up the baby. I welcomed extended time on the sofa in those early days, and I didn't rush to get going, but I found that my body surprised me by how quickly it healed and got used to the new demands. I even went on a ski holiday at four months postpartum (something I've previously done) and I was so scared that my core would let me down, but after a few tentative runs, I felt like the 'old' me! It's a huge challenge for your body to go through, alongside trying to care for your newborn, but I was pleasantly surprised by the speed and extent of the recovery. In hindsight, I didn't need to be so apprehensive, and I'd possibly opt for an elective C-section next time, as I liked how organized and controlled it was.

Having not researched much into C-section or C-section recovery (it wasn't on my plan A, B, or C) it was interesting to see, when I discovered The 360 Mama, that such a recovery was possible. It's easy to think that the 'C-section shelf' is an unavoidable and necessary side-effect of a C-section, but the content on social media, and the approach to the massaging, definitely helped me understand appropriate expectations regarding recovery and appearance. I signed up for the online course within the first few weeks and I liked how it guided you through the different techniques, at different stages of recovery, including appropriate exercises, and the WHY behind the massaging techniques – so important!

Knowing about the different layers of scar tissue helped me come to terms with my scar and understand how to treat it. Not only that, it was so refreshing to hear from other women who also feel like they didn't receive the service they needed from the doctors during their 12-week check/postnatal care. So many women are let down and their concerns brushed aside once the baby has arrived. Knowing that our concerns are valid and having someone invested in our recovery has been invaluable. It just goes to show how crucial the work of The 360 Mama team is and how much it can impact new mums. This course and resources (including this book) have been a vital part of my recovery, and I wish every mum had access to this quality of support and guidance.

22

Types of C-section scars

Everybody who has a C-section will end up with a scar on the outside of their body that will remain forever, however this will look different for each person. You will also have scar tissue below the surface scar, with adhesions between the different layers of tissues that will have been cut through to get to baby (these adhesions can also stick to surrounding organs too) and a scar on your uterus, but no-one can be sure about what could be happening here, or the extent of this scar tissue, without further surgery to look closely at it. We can, however, get an idea of what's going on by assessing the symptoms you're experiencing, and by the movement and feel of the scar and surrounding tissue.

All surgery creates scars and adhesions that cannot be removed entirely (so you will keep that smile on your tummy as a souvenir of your birth). But we can often improve the look of your scar, how it feels to touch, and how the scar and its area feels when you move, as well as the impact it's having on your body.

It's really important to understand the type of scar you have so that you can correctly treat it. Different scar types require different massage techniques and products to improve and treat them, and incorrect treatment could make your symptoms and scar worse. There are also often things you can do prior to your C-section to impact the outcome of your scar, particularly if you are prone to more severe scarring like keloid scars. See Chapter 2 on preparing for a C-section.

Types of scars

The type of scar you have may impact the issues you experience with it, and makes a difference to how you approach your recovery.

Flat line scar
This type of scar is flush with the skin; it will be smooth and flat, it's likely it won't feel tight or be pulled in. It won't be raised above the

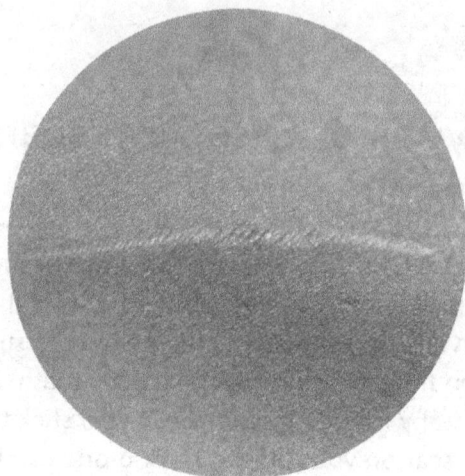

Figure 22.1 Flat line scar

surrounding tissue and can usually easily be lifted with your fingers. It's the least likely scar type to be problematic, but there may still be adhesions in tissues below the scar that can cause concern, so this scar type will still benefit from scar massage.

Hypertrophic

A hypertrophic scar is a scar that is raised and looks like it sits on top of the skin. It's caused by the body over-producing collagen at the scar site during healing. It may be firm, red/purple, rubbery, shiny and look a bit ropey or like a rounded shoelace on your skin. This is different from a keloid scar though, in that the scar itself stays within the border of the scar, so it's often quite smooth looking along the edges.

Keloid

Similar to a hypertrophic scar, a keloid scar happens when your body produces too much collagen during healing except here. The collagen grows to form both a raised scar but also one that grows around the scar too. These scars are firm, raised, rubbery, and also often itchy, painful and can impact your movement (although this can be true of all scar tissue, especially when you have adhesions below the surface).

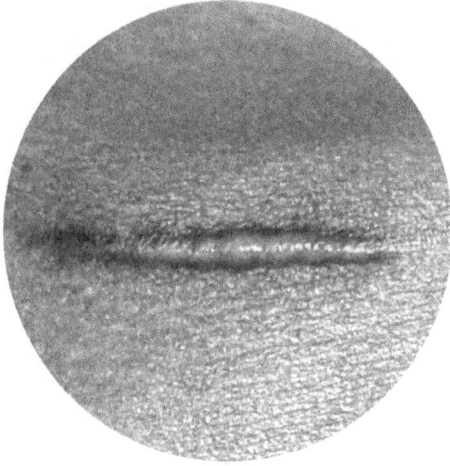

Figure 22.2 Hypertrophic scar

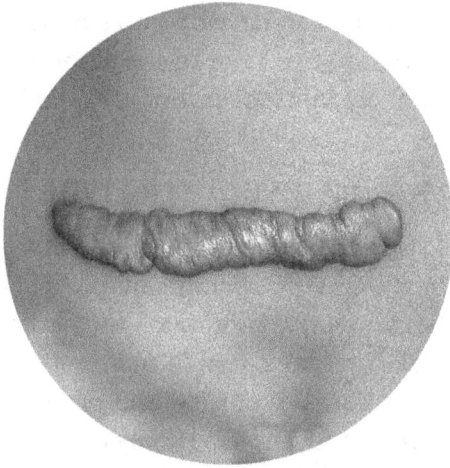

Figure 22.3 Keloid scar

Widespread or atrophic

This type of scar will usually have a sunken, indented appearance, and the scar itself may be quite wide. This happens when the body can't regenerate tissue properly, and in the case of C-section scars is usually due to an infection after your C-section surgery or slow, poor healing.

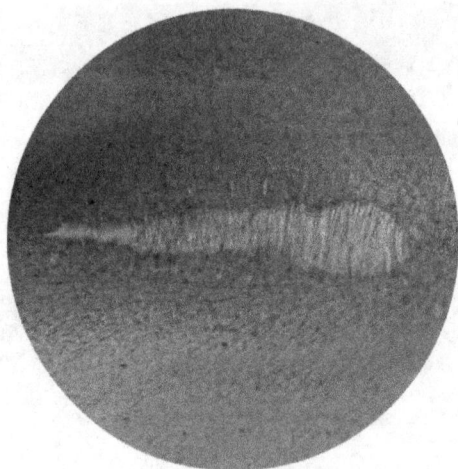

Figure 22.4 Widespread scar

Scars that are left untreated can develop into a hypertrophic or keloid scar even months after surgery, so it's really important to correctly treat your scar with appropriate massage techniques and products.

Things to know about your scar type

As your wound heals and the scar forms, it may go through stages of being a variety of these types of scar. Different parts of your scar can also be different scar types whilst it goes through the healing and maturing process (which can take up to two years), and even years later.

How your scar looks from the outside isn't necessarily an indication of how it's affecting your body, as this is only one part of the scar tissue created during the operation. We need to consider all of the layers involved in the operation, and all scars can benefit from treatment with massage and scar products.

Keloid scars are more likely to occur in people of certain ethnicities and with darker-coloured skin. People of South Asian, Chinese, African Caribbean or Black African origin are more likely to develop these types of scars. However, they can occur on any skin type or colour.

If you already have a keloid or hypertrophic scar elsewhere on your body, this is a good indication that your C-section scar is likely to do the same. This is because your body's healing process tends to be consistent across different injuries.

Trauma can also really impact scar formation and may be a result of physical trauma from an invasive C-section surgery, excessive tension on the wound site during healing, an infection, or slow recovery of the wound. Emotional trauma can also affect your body's ability to heal well, so addressing any emotional birth trauma can be really important for a good physical recovery of your wound.

It's particularly important with keloid and hypertrophic scars not to overstimulate or pull on them with certain massage techniques, as it could increase the production of collagen.

Even if you are more prone to a certain scar type it isn't necessarily a certainty, and each person's healing process is unique. We go into depth about different treatments for each scar type in Chapter 11 (scar products) and Chapter 24 (scar massage), so make sure you read those before beginning to massage your scar.

23

What causes the C-section overhang or shelf?

Nearly everyone believes or has been told that their C-section overhang is due to weight gain and can only be 'treated' by losing it. This simply isn't true: people of all sizes can experience an overhang, and we have treated very slim women with large overhangs as well as plus-sized women without them. A frustration we hear all the time from clients after they get back to their pre-baby weight, is that they still have an overhang, confirming it was not their weight that was causing it. At this point, many women are led to believe there is nothing that can be done, or that they would need to resort to more surgery such as a tummy tuck to change the appearance of their overhang.

If the appearance of your overhang does not bother you, and you do not struggle with pulling, tightness or potential skin issues or infections under the shelf, then it is not necessarily a problem that you need to treat. How you feel about your postpartum body is very personal, and while it's wonderful to embrace the changes you see after birth, it's also absolutely fine to not feel that way. We particularly advocate treating your scar because we know it is often the cause of many physical issues too, but wanting to improve the appearance of your overhang is a very valid concern as well. Understanding what it is and what causes it will give you more options for how to treat it.

There are over ten different reasons that you may have an overhang after a C-section, and any number of them could apply to you. Below we are going to explain what these are, why they could be causing your overhang and what you can do to resolve them.

An overhang is one of the main things women come to us for help with. It can be really challenging to see this change in your body following a C-section, especially if it wasn't expected. Due to the multiple reasons for your having had a C-section, and how long it takes for your body to recover, an overhang is always the last thing to go, which can be really frustrating, but trust the process. C-section overhangs can often be completely treated, and if not, greatly improved.

Why you may have an overhang

Scar tissue

Scar tissue can cause adhesions. This is when your scar and the tissues below it that have also been cut through stick to each other and often create a pulled in-looking scar. If your scar is tight and locked down, this can mean that your tummy above it (even if it's a very slim tummy) often hangs over the top of the scar as the stuck-down scar creates a shelf. By massaging your C-section scar and using products to hydrate and soften the scar tissue, you can help to reduce these adhesions creating a flatter, less pulled-in scar, and therefore a flatter-appearing abdomen.

Swelling

It is really normal for swelling to occur after surgery. This inflammation phase is a normal part of the healing process and the medication used during an C-section operation as well as postpartum hormones can cause swelling. When your abdomen is swollen above your scar this can make your scar look more pulled in and exaggerate your overhang. For some women, a degree of swelling may hang around after the acute healing phase has finished and your lymphatic system just needs a helping hand to get rid of this. This may appear as puffy or spongy skin above or below your scar. Good hydration and nutrition is essential here but light, pumping massage techniques can really help the body to eliminate this waste product, helping to create a flatter appearance to your tummy. We cover these massage techniques in the scar massage chapter.

Diastasis recti (tummy separation)

This could be creating a more rounded appearance to your abdomen. This occurs when the connective tissue that bridges the gap between the left and right side of the abdominal wall is stretched and thinned during pregnancy as your bump grows and the muscles separate. Sometimes after you've given birth that tissue does not regain its original shape or strength, meaning the left and right side remain separated, and so the tummy has a bloated appearance. Weakness in your tummy muscles could also be contributing to your overhang if you do not rehabilitate the deep core muscles which encourage the tummy to draw back in after birth. In both cases the pressure in the abdomen will bulge outwards against the weaker tissue of the abdominal wall and affect the appearance of your midsection and overhang.

Weak core muscles

Often we find women are gripping their upper abdominal or oblique muscles (sides of the abdomen) through stress or from poor posture or bad habits and repetitive actions such as slouching or flexing the trunk while feeding. This causes a compressive force around the upper abdomen, forcing pressure downwards, which creates the appearance of a pouch in the lower abdomen. This is especially noticeable if the lower abs are weaker. Learning to re-engage your deep core more effectively can help to change the appearance and function of your stomach. In this scenario, you'll need to not only strengthen the lower ab area, but also improve the mobility in the trunk higher up and retrain your core to let go of some bad habits. You'll see this demonstrated in the exercise plan laid out in Chapter 25 and Chapter 26.

Hydration

When you're dehydrated, your body holds on to water, which can make you look swollen. Good hydration is also essential for good scar healing. When breastfeeding, be particularly mindful to increase your water intake.

Nutrition

You need plenty of protein and vitamins, minerals and energy for your body and tummy to heal well. The best way to ensure you are giving your body what it needs is to eat a healthy diet. We cover this in more detail in Chapter 8, but typically you'll want to increase your protein intake for collagen production and repairing and building new tissue, as well as helping to maintain muscle strength. Vitamin C is vital for producing collagen, so you should ensure your diet is plentiful in vegetables and fruit that have a high index, or you could consider taking supplements.

The early days of recovery are not the time to be trying to lose your baby weight. You'll need plenty of carbohydrates for energy and to support breast milk production if you choose to breastfeed your baby. You may also need to address your iron levels if you suffered blood loss during your birth. This can often be supported by a good diet, but if you are worried you can ask your doctor to do a blood test to check your iron levels and in some cases a supplement may be advised.

It's very important to keep your gut healthy and functioning well in the weeks after birth. Medication and the impact of abdominal surgery can make your bowels behave differently, and you really want to avoid episodes of constipation as you recover, as this can be very painful and also cause more strain for your pelvic floor, increasing your risk of pelvic floor problems. Iron tablets can typically cause constipation, so if you do require them, you'll want to be extra mindful of how you can support good gut health and bowel health with your diet and by maintaining good hydration levels.

Hernia

This can occur as a result of changes to your body during pregnancy or as a result of surgery itself.

There are different types of hernia. Following a C-section, it is possible for an incisional hernia to occur where the lining of your abdomen or organs behind it escape through the incision from your C-section where the tissue is weaker. This is a rare complication, but you can reduce the risk by resting appropriately and avoiding doing things like lifting, pushing or anything with excess force while you heal. Some signs and symptoms of an incisional hernia are:

- Pain and swelling at the site of your incision
- A bulge you can see and feel at the incision site
- Constipation, vomiting or feeling unwell. These symptoms can occur in more serious cases where the hernia becomes strangulated, affecting the blood flow to your bowel, so you should seek medical advice as soon as possible.

This type of hernia should not be confused with an 'overhang', although it may present as a bulging of the scar.

Other types of postpartum hernias include umbilical hernia at the belly button, hiatal hernia in the upper abdomen, or less frequently an inguinal hernia in the groin. A hernia in the abdomen (umbilical or hiatal) may occur as a result of the stretching of the connective tissue in pregnancy, causing it to be weaker, and can be associated with diastasis recti as discussed above.

Some common signs of an umbilical hernia are:

- A 'new' outy belly button or change of appearance at your belly button
- A bulge in the abdominal wall
- Repetitive bloating or abdominal discomfort.

While these issues are a separate condition, they can indicate some dysfunction of the abdominal and core muscles, which can in turn affect the appearance of your tummy and create more of an overhang.

If you are concerned about a hernia, you should get it checked by your doctor. You may require a surgical repair, although this is unlikely to be offered too soon after a C-section. For some people, hernias don't cause any symptoms or problems and can be managed well without surgery, but it's always best to get it checked.

Loose skin

It's normal to have loose skin and stretch marks after pregnancy, particularly on your abdomen. This can improve with time, good hydration (internally and with hydrating skin products), nutrition and movement, but this is one factor that is particularly hard to eliminate. Although you may be left with loose skin, treating the other issues that could be causing your overhang can still make an improvement to your overhang.

Stress and lack of sleep

Stress and lack of sleep can cause your body to hold on to fat around your middle as the body behaves as if it is in 'survival mode' and slows down your recovery. Poor sleep and fatigue can also increase inflammation in the body and therefore more swelling. While we know that most mothers will struggle with poor sleep with a new baby, it's another reminder to rest when you can, and not feel guilty about prioritizing it over other tasks.

Tummy fat

This is totally normal post-birth, and weight loss can't be 'targeted' to any particular area with any diet or exercise plan despite what you might read. Losing weight will of course reduce the size of your abdomen, which will contribute to a flatter-appearing scar, but without addressing the other factors above, this alone won't be the solution to treating your overhang.

As you can see, there are lots of ways to address your overhang, most of which are simple changes you can make from home. Being aware of these things ahead of time may help you to plan some parts of your recovery, but it's really important to say that it's also never too late to start treating your scar and the overhang.

24

C-section scar massage

What is scar massage?

Scar massage is a way of improving the way your scar looks, how it feels and how it's affecting your body. There are a number of issues (mentioned below) that your scar could be causing or contributing to, and scar massage can help alleviate these too.

It can help to soften and flatten scars and improve things like pain and tension, an overhang, and how you feel about your scar and body following surgery. During the first six months after surgery, your body's priority at the wound site is laying down collagen as quickly as possible to close the wound. The collagen is laid down in a mish-mash formation, which can often mean the area is tough, dense and immobile.

It's thought that by massaging your scar during this period you can help this mess of scar tissue heal in a more organized formation, meaning the scar tissue moves better and works better with the surrounding tissue, causing fewer issues. However, this doesn't mean that once you've reached six months post-birth you can no longer affect and improve scar tissue. The connective tissue of your body is constantly reshaping itself, so it's possible to loosen scar adhesions and improve elasticity even years later, so it's absolutely worth massaging your scar even if it's been years since you gave birth.

Scar massage never needs to hurt and we certainly don't want to be causing additional trauma to the area, which can slow down the healing process and potentially cause more scar tissue. It's just about getting the tissues moving, and you don't need to spend more than five to ten minutes a day doing it to see an improvement.

Why do you need to massage your C-section scar?

In order to birth your baby abdominally, layers of tissue (skin, fascia, nerves and muscle) have been pulled apart or cut through. A scar forms in each of these layers to close these incisions; an essential part of healing. However, scar tissue is a lot more dense, thick and tough than 'normal' tissue, and likes to stick to surrounding tissues, often causing adhesions (scar tissue that sticks to surrounding organs). Not only can this new scar tissue and adhesions cause issues such as restrictions, tension, pain and pulling at the scar area itself but, where the adhesions stick to their surroundings, it can also cause issues globally throughout your body. Lots of people also experience heightened sensitivity around the scar and/or numbness following the surgery.

It's common that the build-up of scar tissue can cause your tummy to protrude or 'overhang'. We often see clients with a band of thick, lumpy scar tissue just above their C-section scar, which then sits over their scar. Many clients also find that the area around their scar or the scar itself feels hard or immobile, and when thick tissue is held down like this, it's common for your tummy to then hang over the top of it.

Swelling is also often seen after a C-section. This is a normal part of healing in the early stages, but for some women this 'puffiness' around their scar remains for months after, and needs a helping hand to move it out of the body.

Left untreated, scar tissue can contribute to common issues such as back pain, hip pain, incorrect breathing patterns, constipation, pelvic floor issues, urinary urgency, deep thrusting pain during sex as well as pelvic pain. Sometimes these issues will appear quite soon after birth, but it's not uncommon for them to come on months or even years after surgery; it's never too late to make a difference to your scar and the problems it may cause.

Lots of clients come to us unable to look at or touch their scars. This is such a normal response, especially if you weren't expecting to have a C-section (as many people aren't), if you had a traumatic birth, or just didn't get the birth you had hoped for. Often when we hold on to trauma or have negative associations with an area of our body, the brain disassociates with that area. When you feel completely disconnected from your abdominal area and core after pregnancy, it's unrealistic to expect it to work well when you need it in real life or during exercise. Speaking to someone about your experience is really important to heal, but touch is also incredibly important to fully recover. Massage can help you reconnect with the area and come to terms with your birth, but it's also important to not disassociate from your abdominal area. If you are disconnected from your tummy, it can be hard to engage these muscles properly and could mean the core rehab you're doing may not be very effective, or is hard to perform correctly. Not touching your scar can also mean that issues such as itching, numbness and sensitivity persist, but by touching the area you can re-establish the nerve connection and resolve or lessen them. We find that the sooner clients touch the area, the quicker normal sensation returns, and they experience less numbness, hypersensitivity or itching.

It's totally understandable after major abdominal surgery to be wary of the area and concerned that massaging it can cause damage or that it will hurt, but as long as your wound is completely closed over and you go gently, it's very unlikely that this would be the case.

Clients who come to us for scar treatment often come expecting scar massage to be unpleasant, when in actual fact most find it relaxing and enjoyable. They leave feeling more connected with, and accepting of, their scar, and the incredible journey their body has been through.

Benefits of scar massage

Although your scar isn't the only reason you may be experiencing the issues below, if you have ruled out other explanations with your doctor, it's possible your scar is contributing to or causing these problems. Scar massage can help:

- Reduce pain
- Improve your overhang
- Reduce tension
- Improve digestive issues
- Improve heavy periods
- Improve other issues such as shoulder pain, headaches, migraines, TMJ (jaw) pain
- Improve incontinence
- Improve chronic neck/hip lower back pain
- Improve constipation
- Improve itching
- Improve the look and feel of the scar itself – less red, raised and flatter

- Stimulate the nerves that have been cut during the operation. This can reduce pain, numbness, sensitivity and itching
- Help you to reconnect with your tummy muscles. This can improve any tummy muscle separation, improve posture and core strength, help to reduce hip and back pain and improve pelvic floor function, getting you feeling more like yourself again
- Soften and release scar tissue. This can improve the appearance and overhang of the scar and reduce pulling around it. It can also release the scar from the tissues below and organs, improve any bladder or bowel issues, reduce any pain during intercourse and possibly improve the chances of conceiving again – if you want to!

Do's and don'ts

- You can actually begin scar massage from day one post-birth by using diaphragmatic breathing. This will gently mobilize and massage the scar tissue from the inside out, encourage the scar tissue to lay down in a more organized way, speed up healing and help prevent adhesions to the tissues below.
- Placing your hands flat and lightly over your scar through clothes to perform your diaphragmatic breathing at this time will also help to restore sensation and help you reconnect with the area.
- Hands-on massage can be applied, from as little as 1–2 weeks after surgery, but only above the scar and very lightly. Gently brushing your hands over your abdomen and towards the scar can help encourage healing and help restore sensation, but avoid the incision site itself at this stage. From 6–8 weeks – and as long as your scar is fully healed, closed over and scab free, you can massage directly over your scar. Start really lightly with brushing strokes to begin with.
- You can massage your scar with an oil if you prefer, but we find that most techniques work better performed on dry skin without an oil as you can get better mobility through the layers of tissues, then you can apply the oil after you have massaged.

- There are some oils and creams you can apply from day one and some from week two (please see Chapter 11) that can really speed up the healing process and improve the outcome of your scar. Make sure your hands are clean and dry before applying these and just gently dab the product along the scar in these early days.
- You only need to spend around five to ten minutes a day massaging your scar to see results, and massaging for extended periods or too often may cause more harm than good.
- If it hurts when you're massaging your scar or the surrounding area, or after you've massaged your scar, it's likely that you're doing it too hard.
- Do massage your full abdomen, your scar and all around your scar for best results.

What if you can't touch your scar?

If this is you, please know that this is really common, and that it doesn't need to be a barrier to scar massage. From all the clients we've treated in person who've had this issue, all of them have been pleasantly surprised by how OK they were with us massaging their scars, and have walked out of our sessions together feeling so much more confident about touching and massaging their scars themselves. It really is possible to overcome this, especially as you do not need to touch your scar at all to begin scar massage.

Below we go through the stages of how to begin scar massage, and although some of these are aimed at the early days of healing, we would advise you start from the very beginning if you are wary about touching your scar. Begin with your breathwork, and light touch around and towards the scar, and you can absolutely do this through clothes to make it less worrying. As you start to feel more confident to move closer to the scar itself, you can perform the massage techniques through clothes or by using objects or massage tools. A lot of people also find it easier for someone else to touch it first, so you may want to ask your partner to have a read through this chapter and try out some of the gentle starting techniques to see how it feels with them doing the massage before you give it a try yourself.

If you are unable to progress to touching your scar, we would recommend requesting your birth stories from the hospital to help process any trauma that may be holding you back, or seeking help from a birth trauma practitioner (see Chapter 18). You may also find it easier to have an in-person scar massage treatment with a professional first to give you the confidence to touch your scar.

Scar massage

Scar massage doesn't only mean massaging the scar you can see: the whole tummy area (and your body) can be affected by the surgery. The cuts that have been made internally are usually made above the scar you can see, so you may have lumpy scar tissue above your scar or stuck dense tissue around the scar. So it's always beneficial to massage around the scar too.

Where to begin

Before you do any kind of massage, simply placing your hands on your tummy and possibly over your scar site (very gently and through clothes) is a great way to just reconnect with the area. We would advise doing this as regularly as you can from the very start.

Diaphragmatic breathing

As we've mentioned in the do's and don'ts, this is the best place to start massaging your C-section scar and the surrounding area. And it's great because you can use it from day one post-birth. This is a fantastic way to get the area moving gently, which can really help to speed up healing and get the scar tissue moving early on, helping to potentially limit adhesions and issues with your scar.

Video: Diaphragmatic Breathing Tutorial #1

Light touch away from the scar

This technique can again be used from a few days post-birth, when you feel ready to touch your abdomen. If you have any bruising or a lot of pain, it's best to wait until this has eased before beginning. However, this is a very light technique that will help promote healing in the area, restore sensation and treat issues such as numbness or hypersensitivity and itching, and help you to reconnect with the area.

We would recommend trying this technique through a thin piece of clothing first. With a flat, soft hand, slowly and lightly brush your hand down from your ribs in the direction of your scar but don't yet go over the scar itself. The pressure should feel like you're lightly stroking. You can also do this around your hips towards your scar and up your upper legs towards your scar too. Once you feel OK with this through clothes you can progress to applying this directly skin on skin.

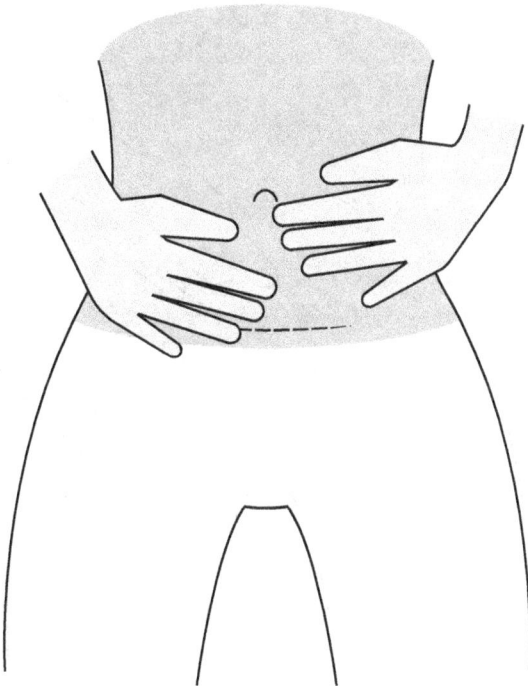

Figure 24.1 Gentle stroking with flat hands towards the C-section scar promotes healing

Using 'tools'

Touching and massaging the scar area and around it with soft objects is a great way to start massaging your scar. This is perfect for clients who don't feel like they can touch the area directly, to introduce touch and build up to working directly with hands. Light touch is fantastic for calming down or stimulating the nerves in the area, so this is also a good technique if you're struggling with numbness or hypersensitivity. Many clients do at the start (it's common for this to continue for months/years after too if left untreated). Your nerves respond well to different textures and temperatures (we love using the back of a spoon from the fridge and gently gliding it over the skin) so mixing up what you're using will really help to improve sensation by getting those nerve endings firing correctly again.

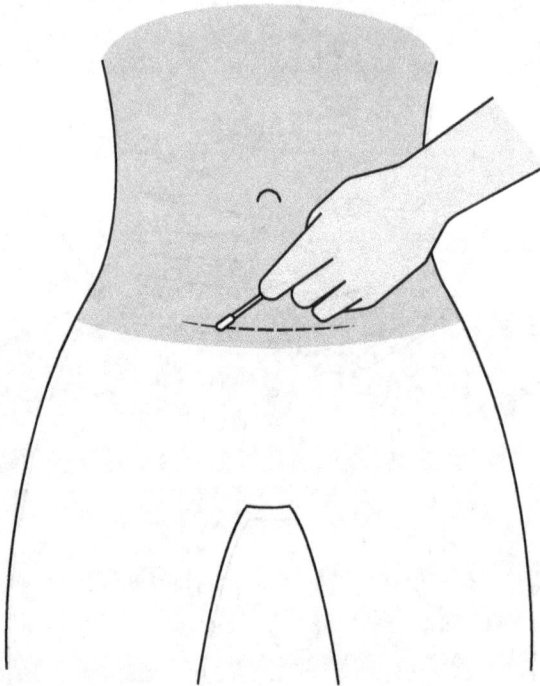

Figure 24.2 Touching the scar with soft objects such as a cotton bud helps stimulate the nerves and promotes healing

Grab yourself a range of tools you can easily find around the house. Examples include:

- A new clean make-up brush
- Cotton wool
- Cotton wool bud
- A small ball
- A soft scarf
- The back of a metal spoon
- A super soft toothbrush, or baby hairbrush.

Starting above the scar and working over your full abdomen, slowly brush the tools all over your tummy in lots of different directions. You can mix up the speed with more of a fast zigzag motion to help stimulate the nerve endings but keep the pressure light. If your scar is fully healed, you can do this over your scar as well, with clean objects.

Hypertrophic/keloid scars

Scars that are red and raised, such as hypertrophic or keloid scars, are like this due to the body producing excess collagen at the scar site. We don't want to encourage this further by overstimulating these types of scars. As such, any fast, vigorous techniques should be avoided over the scar itself if it looks like this.

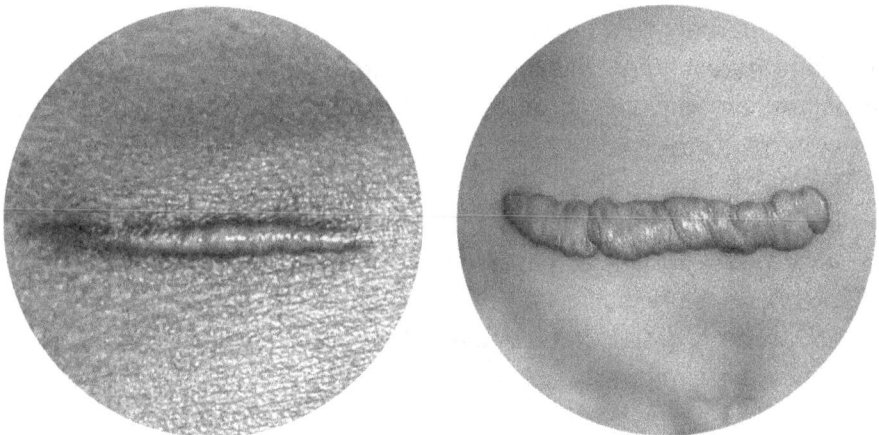

Figure 24.3 Keloid and hypertrophic scars

How to massage your scar

Once you've reached 6–8 weeks postpartum and your scar is fully healed, you can begin scar massage over the actual scar. If you are at all unsure whether your scar is ready, please speak to your doctor before beginning, and stick to the above techniques until you've done so. The techniques we use to massage the scar are light and gentle, you don't need to dig around in there – that could potentially make recovery take even longer if you are causing more trauma to the area.

The easiest position, we find, to massage your scar in reclined on the sofa or propped up in bed so you can see what you're doing whilst also having a relaxed abdomen. However, anything is better than nothing, and if you find that doing it in the bath or shower is the only time you're getting it done, that's totally fine.

We find that massaging without an oil is best to get more mobility in your scar, particularly with certain techniques where we are trying to get a grip on the skin and create mobility between the layers. Apply your oil after you've done your massage.

Aim for five to ten minutes a day of massage.

When not to massage your scar

If you are experiencing any of the below then massage is not appropriate for your scar right now:

- If you are prior to six weeks postpartum
- If you have a fungal infection or a rashes
- If you have any scabs or open parts to your scar (it needs to be fully closed)
- If it hurts
- If it's making you feel ill
- In pregnancy – lightly massaging an oil in to your scar if you're pregnant can help alleviate itching and tension in your scar as your tummy grows, but it's advisable to avoid more specific deeper massage techniques.

Three techniques to get you started

Zigzagging technique

We love this for treating nerve issues such as numbness or sensitivity, and for gently introducing touch.

For this technique you want to use one, two or three fingers. The fewer you use, the lighter this technique will be. Most of your nerve endings are in the top, more superficial layers of your skin, so actually the lighter you go with this technique, the better it works on issues such as sensitivity and numbness, but play around with different numbers of fingers and see how this feels for you. You want to keep your fingers straight and flat, then with a nice loose wrist, move in a zigzag pattern over any numb or sensitive areas of your abdomen and all over your scar. Try to focus on an area and move slowly around your abdomen rather than zooming all over the place. You can use your other hand to brace your tummy to help if you have a larger tummy, or even to just be more specific with the technique.

Useful for: Sensitivity or numbness over your scar and abdomen and for smoothing the appearance of your scar, including any stitch or staple marks. It's a great one to use in earlier healing too, so around 6–8 weeks.

Avoid: This technique is not advised over hypertrophic or keloid scars, as it's likely to stimulate the scar to produce more collagen and potentially

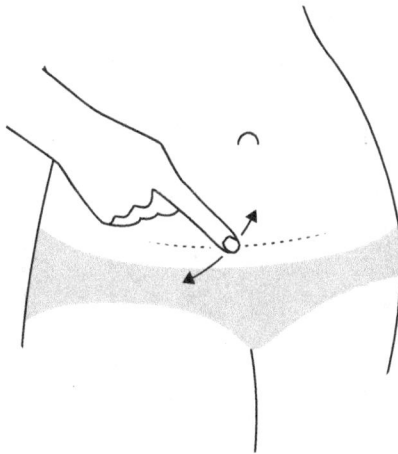

Figure 24.4 Zigzagging technique

worsen the scar. You can use it over any numb or sensitive areas above and away from the scar though, to treat those issues.

Circular dragging technique (without oil)

We love this for a scar that feels stuck down and tight, and for creating a flatter appearance.

Place two fingers on your scar with very little pressure (so you shouldn't be sinking into the scar), and without moving your fingers from that point on your skin, focus on moving and dragging the upper layers of skin and scar tissue around in a circular motion. Repeat this along the full length of the scar from one end to the other, then back again. You can also do this in a dragging motion from side to side along the length of the scar and forwards and backwards over the scar too. The aim here is to get more mobility to the area, so you don't want to be sliding your fingers over your scar, and you should see the scar moving as you do this. You can use this technique (like you can with all of these) all over your abdomen, too. Often we see clients who have a bit of a stuck-down panel of skin above or below their scars – this is a great technique to use on those areas, too.

Useful for: Unsticking the scar from the tissues below, creating more mobility in the scar, helping to incorporate the scar into the surrounding tissue, treating pain and to reduce a pulled in appearance.

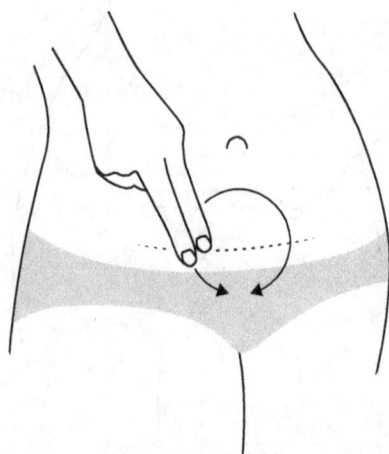

Figure 24.5 Circular dragging technique

Sinking technique

We love this for softening hard, lumpy scar tissue below the scar.

This is a technique we like and give to almost every client as homecare. It's really easy to do and effective on all scar types. See below for a slight adaptation for keloid scars.

With a straight, flat, light and relaxed finger, press and sink into the scar slowly and mindfully, then release the pressure. You can also use this technique through your abdomen as well to soften any scar tissue around the scar (use two or three fingers when doing this). Imagine you're slowly pressing down a button on a keyboard. Work from one end of the scar to the other, spending more time on any harder or lumpier parts.

If your scar is sunken in and feels like it is lacking tissue (like it's missing tissue below it), then you can angle your pressure from the edges of the scar towards the middle to help fill it in and plump it up, creating a flatter appearance.

As long as you work slowly, you can go quite deep with this technique into the tissue/scar, but nothing should be painful or leave it feeling irritated afterwards. If you are finding this painful, you need to warm the area with some lighter techniques first, like the zigzagging technique, or build up to using a deeper pressure.

Useful for: Softening lumpy areas of your scar and hard scar tissue above and below it. This technique can improve any sensitivity you're

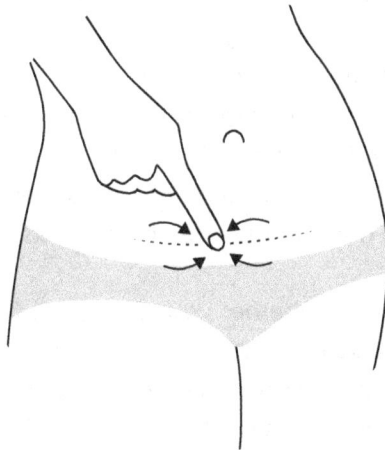

Figure 24.6 Sinking technique

experiencing. The pumping action is also great for reducing swelling around the scar, particularly in an overhang, and helping to improve the movement between layers of scar tissue.

Avoid: For hypertrophic or keloid scars, focus on the edges of the raised scar, pressing from the centre of the scar and sinking off the sides of it, to help incorporate the scar into the surrounding tissue. Spend longer on the more firm parts.

Questions we often get asked about scar massage

Do I need to massage my scar forever?

No, you don't need to massage your scar every day from now on – it is in fact quite hard to say how long you do need to massage it for. As a guide, the purpose of scar massage is to make your scar feel hopefully look better, so if you notice the issues you've been experiencing have subsided, you probably don't need to massage your scar anymore. So just massage it until it feels better. You might notice that once your initial symptoms have subsided, you notice them returning at certain times of the month, so you may want to use the massage techniques then if this happens to help alleviate them. As your scar is maturing for two years post-birth, it's likely you will find it changes as time goes on, and you may get periods where you want to massage it again. Use it as you need it and if you find you haven't massaged your scar for ages and haven't even thought about it, that's a good sign that you're done!

Will my scar go back if I don't keep massaging?

It's thought that the reason scar massage is effective is that it helps to promote healing and encourages the scar to lay down tissue in a more organized formation. So as it progresses in its healing, it should only improve. Generally we find that although it's not uncommon for your scar to feel more painful at a certain time of the month or at the end of the day, for example, these issues usually lessen as time goes on, with regular massage.

If you are at all unsure whether your scar is ready for scar massage, please speak to your doctor before beginning. In this chapter we have just touched on a few techniques that we use for scars as it's difficult to explain them properly without videos, which is why we have a full online course with step-by-step short videos demonstrating all the techniques we use in our clinics, and how to adapt them to different scar types and issues.

Other scar treatments

There are a number of other C-section scar treatments available to help improve your scar: steroid injections, use of machines such as the LymphaTouch, R-shock devices, laser therapy, acupuncture, Botox, and taping to name just a few. Different options will suit different scars, and similarly some treatments may be contraindicated due to individual medical history or scar complications. So if you're interested in any of these treatment options, please speak to your medical provider or a qualified physiotherapist.

My birth story

As I prepared for the birth of my baby, I had everything planned out: a water birth, floating candles, fairy lights, a playlist I had already compiled. It was going to be magical. However, four weeks before the baby was due, I rang up the hospital. The baby had not moved all day and I was getting worried. They told me to come in straight away, and as I drove to the hospital I didn't know what to expect. I was immediately hooked up to the machine that monitors the baby's heartbeat and movements, and while I was lying there, not knowing what was happening, I rang my husband to tell him where I was. He left his work immediately and made his way to the hospital. After an hour and a half of being admitted to the hospital, I was in the surgery room, my husband at my side, and 20 minutes later the nurses handed our baby to my husband. It all happened so fast, I wasn't even sure I was awake (thanks to vivid pregnancy dreams that all seemed too real). We were so happy in that moment, not knowing what lay ahead but thankful that the baby was safe and we could finally meet him.

The next few days were a whirlwind of uncertainty as the baby was taken to the NICU and I was left on the ward without a clue about C-section recovery. I had not read anything about having a C-section or prepared for it in any way at all. No one had ever told me what actually happens when you have a C-section – how big the cut is, how much blood you lose, how long the recovery is, nothing. Over the first couple days I was encouraged to start walking and moving around. I can still remember the first time I walked down to the NICU, which is on the other side of the hospital from the wards. I was sure I was going to pass out from the pain but had been told by a nurse that I did not need a wheelchair anymore. I feel like other people who have major surgery are encouraged to rest and recover, but when a woman has a C-section, it's all about recovering as quickly as possible so you can look after your baby.

Compared to others, I have been told, I recovered very quickly and had no issue with the healing of the scar. I had booked a postnatal appointment with a chiropractor before the birth, and when I went to see him, he showed me how to massage my C-section scar, something I had never even heard of before. I had not even dared to touch my scar yet and it felt very strange to have someone else doing so, but I am so grateful that he taught me how to do it. No one else even mentioned massaging the scar, let alone the importance of doing this, not even the doctor at my 6-week check-up. I have since spoken with friends that have had C-sections and they had no idea what I was talking about. I'm not sure about other countries, but my experience in the UK was that there was little support offered to help me with my C-section recovery. When you leave the hospital, you're handed your baby and told not to lift anything too heavy and not to overdo it, but there is no clear guidance on what this even means. If I had to give advice to anyone expecting a baby, I would tell them to read and find out as much as they can about C-sections, even if they're not planning one, as anything can happen and it is always better to be prepared.

25

Exercises to support scar healing

We do recommend introducing exercises to support your C-section scar healing as soon as it is safe to do so (see below). It is useful for improving blood flow to the area, relieving pain and reducing the risk of blood clots after surgery.

A few weeks on from your surgery, these exercises will also really help by gently moving the scar, and preventing adhesions from developing between the layers of tissue that form the scar. This means the scar is less likely to pull or feel tight when you move around doing normal daily activities. Ideally, as a scar forms we want it to mimic the tissue around it as much as possible. By encouraging it to move gently in a variety of directions we can encourage the scar tissue to form in a uniform pattern that will make it behave more like the tissue around it.

A scar that is not stuck down with adhesions, and can move, glide and slide with the surrounding tissue, will be less restrictive, less likely to be painful and less likely to have an overhang. As we discussed in Chapter 22, the way the scar forms plays a significant part in whether you are left with an overhang or not.

It's also important to highlight that many studies have found women who exercise more in the postpartum period are less likely to struggle with postpartum depression or anxiety, and have better energy levels, so this is another reason to encourage a return to movement and exercise safely.

These exercises should be suitable to begin at approximately four weeks after the birth, as long as you have no complications, no infections and your pain is well managed. This will probably coincide with your starting to do more and to be moving about more in your daily life. It's important to recognize that some gentle exercises such as the ones here are likely to be less strenuous on the body than many of your normal daily activities, which is why it's okay to start to include some before six weeks if you feel well.

If you have received medical advice to avoid exercise completely, you should wait for the all-clear before beginning. Remember, everyone will experience healing at a different rate and it's important not to compare yourself to others or expect your recovery to follow a fixed timeline.

If you experience pain during or after doing these exercises, stop and return to try them again a week later.

Elevating your legs by lying on the floor and resting your feet on the wall is a really great way to help resolve swelling or fluid from building in the feet, ankles or in the lower abdomen around your scar.

Connecting with your pelvic floor and deep abdominal muscles

You should have already begun to engage with your pelvic floor in the early exercises mentioned in Chapter 15. Now you've connected with the muscles and feel confident that you're doing the exercises correctly, it's time to gradually increase the challenge.

The technique will be the same (refer to Chapter 15 for video instructions), but progressing to practising doing them in different positions adds more load to the muscles and therefore strengthens them further.

- On all fours
- Sitting
- Side-lying
- Standing.

You may find the exercises harder to do in some positions, but it's important you persevere until you master the technique, as your pelvic floor will have to be able to perform in similar positions in real life. You should aim to perform ten repetitions of the slow and fast efforts in all these positions.

How exercise can help to reduce a C-section shelf or overhang

Some of the most common issues we see that contribute to an overhang can be improved with exercise. These include:

- Swelling is a normal part of recovering from surgery, but for some people it can take a long time for the excess fluid to leave. There can be many causes for this, but the more swelling you have around or above the scar the more prominent your overhang can appear. Gently introducing exercise that helps to increase blood flow and encourage better lymphatic drainage can ease swelling earlier.
- A lack of mobility in the scar and surrounding tissue. As the scar forms it can often create adhesions to the layers of tissue around it. This means the scar becomes stuck and can form a shelf over which the rest of the abdomen hangs over. By encouraging the scar and surrounding tissue to move at the earliest opportunity, and continue to move as it forms and matures, you can help to prevent this from happening.
- Poor connection to the lower abdominal muscles. This might be as a result of altered sensation and nerve function in the abdomen following surgery, or a lack of rehabilitation to retrain the muscles to activate effectively after pregnancy and birth. Without this, the brain can become disassociated from the area, and the muscles may not recover their previous strength or function.
- Whether through pain, or the demands of early motherhood such as feeding, carrying and holding a baby, your posture can change, meaning you spend more time in positions that cause excess pressure to push into your lower tummy or pelvis. This can create more of a pooching effect as the lower tummy bulges.
- Your C-section scar can also interfere with your pelvic floor function. Since the pelvic floor muscles are an essential part of your lower core strength, a lack of connection to your pelvic floor can affect the appearance of your lower tummy and pooch.

To address the overhang effectively we recommend that exercise be focused on the deep core, lower abdominal muscles, pelvic floor muscles, hip mobility, pelvic stability, gluteal strength and mobility for the upper back to improve posture and diaphragm function. As you can see, for the best results you'll need to take a global approach rather than just focusing on the local area.

Video: Scar and Abdominal Muscle Training Tutorial #1

To follow video instructions of the exercises that follow in this chapter, please use the QR codes to visit our exercise library.

'Upper Body Movements'

These will help to ease postural aches and pains that commonly occur as a result of feeding positions, altered sleeping positions or the effort of carrying and holding a newborn.

2–4 weeks
Supine-lying pec openings
Side-lying arm openings with bent elbow
Crook-lying overhead reach
Crook-lying overhead arm scissors
Full body stretch
Doorway stretch single arm, progress to double

4–6 weeks
Cat stretch, progress to cat/camel
Side-lying arm openings full
Thread needle
Wall press-up
Prone half cobra
Mermaid

Hands on: Scar and Abdominal Muscle Training Tutorial #2
'Lower Body Movements'

These will aid pelvis and core recovery, resolving pain and regaining some early strength to help you cope with the demands of looking after a newborn.

2–4 weeks
Pelvic tilt
Pillow squeeze bridge
Clam pillow squeeze
Quads stretch
Pelvic tilt on all fours
Knee rolls

4–6 weeks
Core engagement with yoga block press in crook-lying
Core engagement with ball press in side-lying
Core engagement with knee to palm press in crook-lying
Hip thrusts
Kneeling hip flexor stretch
Clam
Kneel up

These exercises have been chosen to directly influence your scar recovery and mobility, and provide the foundations for rebuilding your core. This should help to reduce any pain or discomfort you may feel and make day-to-day activities feel easier. For additional exercises with a focus on further core strengthening and preparation for returning to more challenging fitness or exercise, please refer to the next chapter.

26

Exercise for further core strengthening and readiness to return to sport or fitness

This is a progression beyond the previous chapter, and the exercises should be used in that order. If you haven't yet, start your exercise journey from the start of Chapter 25 and work your way through to this point.

This isn't so as to slow your progress, but because if you don't restore your deep core and pelvic floor connection and resolve postural imbalances that affect your form as you exercise, you probably won't get the results you are hoping for when it comes to addressing core strength, and you may still be at risk of injury.

Postpartum return to running guidelines from the UK recommend that running and other impact exercise should not begin until at least 12 weeks after birth. This will vary from person to person, but is a good reminder to not rush your return.

If this is your goal, you must also be aware that you will not be ready to return to sport or fitness classes simply because 12 weeks have passed. To return to pre-pregnancy function, your body will require some rehabilitation, so our recommendation is to use this time to work on rebuilding your strength so that your body is capable and ready to cope with the demands of your chosen sport or fitness routine when the time comes.

These short exercise routines should take five to ten minutes to complete. You don't need to be working out for long sessions during this period of your recovery to achieve your goals. It's unlikely to be feasible anyway with a young baby to care for, but you should also be careful not to deplete your energy stores with lots of exercise when you are still healing, may be sleep deprived, and you'll be using a lot of energy for breastfeeding if you've chosen to.

This is not an exercise programme designed to help you lose weight or to make your body look a certain way. Its purpose is to help you achieve a strong, pain-free body so that you can return to other forms of exercise safely when you've healed. We'd strongly recommend that you do not use this period of your recovery to diet or limit your calorie intake or focus on using exercise for weight loss.

These are just some examples of exercises you could be doing, but it is by no means an exhaustive list. There are many safe options for postpartum exercise, but we do recommend that you ensure you are following programmes from qualified professionals who have a full understanding of the postpartum body, and specifically C-section scar behaviour. If you have been advised by a medical professional that exercise is not suitable for you, or you have any concerns, you should seek the advice of a medical professional before embarking on any exercise programme.

Hands on: Progression Abdominal Muscle Training Tutorial #1

Weeks 4–6
Bridge + ball squeeze
Superman
All fours hover
Thread needle
Scissors
Sideplank
Kneeling press-up
Bridge + march
Side stretch

6–12 weeks mobility
Prone cobra, progress to twist
Bench press up
Row backs

Superman
Band openings
Lunge + thoracic twist

6–12 weeks strength
Scissors
Superman
All fours hip circles
Single leg bridge
Squat to high knee
Standing hip flexor with band
Reverse lunge to high knee
Forward lunge to high knee
Side lunge
Side adductor slides

When you've worked your way through these series of exercises, or your own equivalent postpartum programme and you're feeling well, you can start to think about returning to more general forms of fitness. The purpose of working through movements like this is to ensure that you have a good baseline of strength to tolerate and cope with the demands of more challenging exercise. We'd recommend always trying to include some form of exercise that allows you to consistently work on your core and pelvic floor strength after giving birth, because it is the best way to prevent future injuries or problems.

27

Fertility after a C-section birth

Your maternity care will likely be different with any pregnancy that follows a C-section. In the UK for example, you will be offered appointments with an obstetric doctor alongside your usual midwife-led care. Your doctor will likely want to discuss the options for your next birth, and to address any additional risk factors you may have and consider your birthing history. They will be able to advise whether you are a candidate for a VBAC (vaginal birth after a C-section) or whether another C-section would be best for you and your baby. You can discuss your preferences or concerns about this during your appointment. It is important that you understand all your options and why any medical decisions are necessary. So that you can give informed consent for whatever you choose to do.

We often get asked, 'when is it safe to get pregnant again following a C-section?' Every situation is different, and the answer will depend on your own medical history and is best discussed with a medical professional who has the details of this. There is some general advice that may be helpful, but always remember this will not apply to everyone.

Trigger warning: Regularly we have conversations with families who feel they haven't been given enough information to enable them to fully understand why certain medical decisions were made, or why they may be feeling pressured to make decisions that are not aligned with their birth plans. For this reason, we will now discuss some of the risks and benefits associated with C-section births. This includes statistics and information about immediate and long-term impact of C-section delivery. It's worth bearing in mind that all births do have some associated risks, which are largely mitigated by skilled birth practitioners and medical intervention where required. In some cases, if your medical and birth history indicates it, these risks will be discussed with you at the relevant appointments. If you prefer not to read this section, please skip to the end.

It is recommended to wait a minimum of six months but ideally 12–18 months after a C-section before getting pregnant again. Having a C-section means you will have a scar on your uterus. Your C-section scar may be formed and 'healed' by six months after birth, but it can take up to two years for scars to fully mature and to be strong enough to support another pregnancy and withstand labour. Gemma Clifford, Registered Midwife and Birth Educator advises, 'Getting pregnant less than 6 months after giving birth via a Caesarean can increase your risk for a uterine rupture and other complications. A uterine rupture is an acute life-threatening situation for both mother and child, and can also lead to subsequent secondary infertility.' Statistics suggest the risk is low, at one in 200 women,[8] but it is information that may impact your birthing decisions. The risk of complications in pregnancy increases with every subsequent Caesarean birth. Gemma reports, 'Women with previous Caesarean delivery have increased odds of having placenta previa, placenta accreta (a serious condition that can occur in pregnancy when the placenta grows too deeply into the uterine wall and may lead to severe blood loss after birth), uterine rupture, stillbirth in subsequent pregnancy compared to women with a previous vaginal delivery'.[17]

Scars are only ever going to be approximately 70 per cent as strong as 'normal' tissue, so another benefit of leaving sufficient time between pregnancies will allow the tissue to be in the best possible condition and reduce the risks to both you and baby.

Other complications, such as poor wound healing, underlying health conditions, a high BMI, having had multiple C-sections or the incisions being performed vertically on the skin or uterus, will also increase the risks associated with future pregnancies. You may not always be aware if some of these issues apply to you, so it's always best to speak to your medical team about your own medical history before getting pregnant again to make sure your body is ready for another pregnancy.

Can I treat an old C-section scar while pregnant?

Although it's fine to rub a moisturizing cream into your tummy while pregnant, it is not recommended to apply deeper massage techniques to your scar during pregnancy, so you should wait to introduce this for any previous C-section scars until after you've given birth and any new scars have also healed over.

How many C-sections can I have?

Ultimately it's your body and your decision as to how many babies you choose to have, so this is only ever a recommendation and not a rule. Most medical professionals will advise on a maximum of three C-sections due to the increase in risks involved, in particular the weakening of the uterus due to multiple scars and the increased risk of uterine rupture.

Your medical team is there to support you and make a personalized plan with you, so even if you do have additional risk factors, if you get pregnant earlier than planned or are on your fourth or fifth pregnancy, things can be done to limit the risks, such as:

- Planning for a C-section birth rather than a VBAC (vaginal delivery after C-section)
- Monitoring during labour
- Delivering the baby before 40 weeks to limit the stretching of the uterus.

If you do find yourself pregnant earlier than six months post-C-section, or on your fourth or more pregnancy, please don't panic. Book an appointment to discuss it with your medical provider and they will be able to help you make a plan of action. Although the statistics, and risk factors can sound frightening, they are still relatively uncommon and it's likely that your birth team will choose to monitor your pregnancy more closely and put plans in place to support a successful pregnancy and safe birth.

Fertility after C-section

Gemma Clifford, Registered Midwife and Birth Educator, offers some advice about how a C-section birth may affect your future fertility, and highlights some relevant information from current research.

'Women who had undergone a Caesarean section had a 10.6 per cent lower subsequent pregnancy rate. Internal scarring from a C-section can cause obstructions and inflammation in the abdomen and reproductive organs that, in turn, can prevent future pregnancies. This can include intra-abdominal adhesions, fallopian-type dysfunction and uterine abnormalities caused by the Caesarean scar. The inability to conceive after already delivering a child is known as secondary infertility.

Caesarean section can result in an indentation of the uterine muscle (myometrium) at the site of the Caesarean scar, called a niche. When a build-up of fluid occurs at the site it can reduce implantation and cause a toxic environment for an embryo, therefore impacting successful pregnancy.'[18]

In addition to extra scar tissue, a C-section can cause other complications that may determine your fertility fate in the future. Some examples of complications that can arise after a Caesarean include:

- Internal infections at the incision site
- Endometriosis (where tissue similar to that which usually line the womb grow elsewhere)
- Haemorrhages (significant blood loss) from surgery
- Blocked or damaged fallopian tubes
- Defective ovulation and/or irregular menstrual cycles.

Risks and benefits of having a C-section

When making decisions about your birth preferences, you may want to consider some of the pros and cons of C-section birth versus vaginal birth.

Pros	Cons
Caesarean delivery is associated with a reduced rate of urinary incontinence and pelvic organ prolapse compared with long-term outcomes following vaginal delivery, but is not an absolute prevention method.[10]	Be aware of the association with increased risks of outcomes that may affect fertility and future pregnancy. There is limited evidence that children born by C-section may have a higher risk of childhood asthma up to the age of 5 and obesity up to the age of 12.

This information should be given at all points of your pregnancy and healthcare appointments to allow you to make a fully informed decision for birth.

It's also valid to make decisions about your birth preferences based on previous experiences, physical or psychological concerns. Your birth team should listen to your questions and preferences and support you if medically safe to do so.

As a midwife I often recommend the BRAIN acronym as a useful tool for making choices about childbirth and birth planning. It is a logical approach to help you talk through all available options throughout your pregnancy and your birth with your doctor and/or midwife.

What does BRAIN stand for?

- **Benefits** – What are the benefits of making this decision?
- **Risks** – What are the risks associated with this decision?
- **Alternatives** – Are there any alternatives?
- **Intuition** – How do I feel? What does my 'gut' tell me?
- **Nothing** – What if I decide to do nothing/wait and see? What happens next?

Using the information in this chapter to prepare, and having conversations with your medical team, you should now feel better informed to help you make some choices. This is also why it's really important to consider the possibility of a C-section birth even if you are hoping or planning for a vaginal delivery, because birth is often unpredictable. Knowing what your options are and making choices that are well thought out ahead of time can help you to feel a sense of control and calm. In the case of an emergency or crash C-section, it is frequently the loss of control that can trigger negative feelings or trauma afterwards.

Notes for BRAIN planning and questions for your birth team

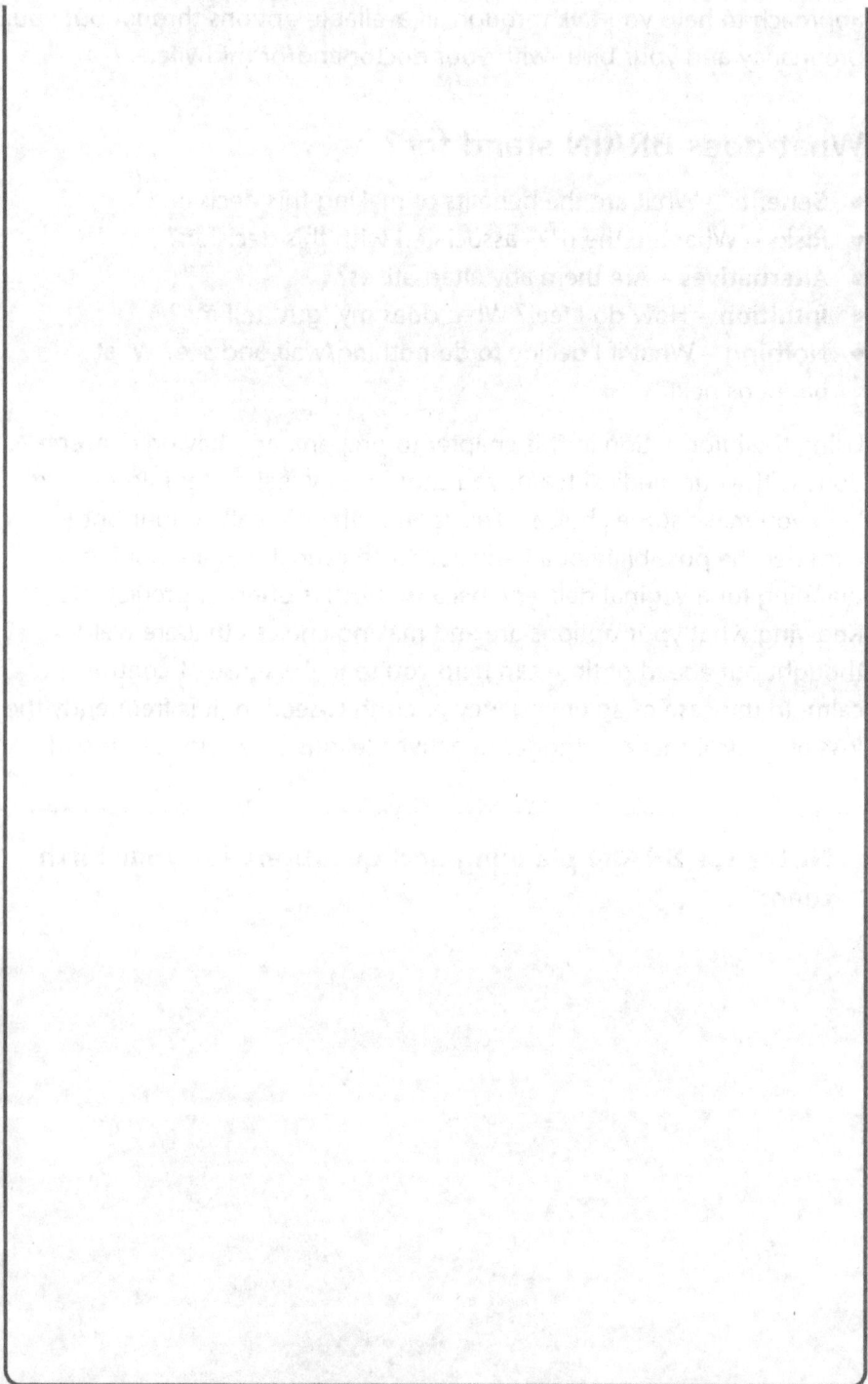

Resources

The 360 Mama International
the360mama.com/

Pelvic Obstetric Gynaecological Physiotherapy, patient information resources
thepogp.co.uk/patient_information/default.aspx

Mummy MOT Clinician Directory UK
www.themummymot.com/for-mums/certified-mummy-mot-practitioners/

Squeezy App Pelvic Health Physio Directory UK (NHS and Private)
squeezyapp.com/directory/

Scar Therapist Directory UK
scarwork.uk/find-a-therapist/

Hannah Poulton Directory UK
https://www.hlp-therapy.co.uk/practitioner-finder

Pelvic Global Directory International
pelvicglobal.com/login/

Pelvic Rehab (USA) – to find a pelvic health practitioner
pelvicrehab.com/

Academy of Pelvic Health Physical Therapy (USA) – their website has a
directory where you can locate a PT near you:
www.aptapelvichealth.org/ptlocator/

Birth Trauma Association
www.birthtraumaassociation.org/

PANDAs for Postnatal Depression
pandasfoundation.org.uk/

Mind for perinatal mental health problems
www.mind.org.uk/information-support/types-of-mental-health-problems/
postnatal-depression-and-perinatal-mental-health/

Tommy's
www.tommys.org/pregnancy-information/im-pregnant/mental-health-wellbeing/postnatal-depression-pnd

My Expert Midwife
myexpertmidwife.com/blogs/my-expert-midwife/c-section-advice-fathers

NCT
www.nct.org.uk/labour-birth/different-types-birth/caesarean-birth/caesarean-birth-recovery-and-practicalities

La Leche
laleche.org.uk/

The Breastfeeding Network
www.breastfeedingnetwork.org.uk/

Pelvic Organ Prolapse
www.pelvicangel.net/

Pelvic Roar
www.pelvicroar.org/

Postpartum Return to Running Guideline
absolute.physio/wp-content/uploads/2019/09/returning-to-running-postnatal-guidelines.pdf

Black Maternal Health (USA)
blackmamasmatter.org/
blackmaternalhealthcaucus-underwood.house.gov/

Black Maternal Health (UK)
fivexmore.org/

C-section recovery hacks

We share daily tips and support across all our social channels, so we thought it would be nice to include some links to some of our videos that might make your C-section recovery a little easier.

To watch our videos please use the QR codes provided below.

Driving home from hospital

www.tiktok.com/@the360mama/video/7264660560262745376

Coughing/sneezing

vm.tiktok.com/ZGeT9VMKq/

Sleeping

vm.tiktok.com/ZGeT9aABG/

Passing your first poo

vm.tiktok.com/ZGeT9Ass8/

Moving around tips

vm.tiktok.com/ZGeT9AEjj/

Getting out of bed

vm.tiktok.com/ZGeT95Cj8/

Showering after a C-section

vm.tiktok.com/ZGeT9uS6R/

Trapped wind

vm.tiktok.com/ZGeT9nVgE/

Constipation

www.tiktok.com/@the360mama/video/7159273267155520773

Contributors

Laura Batten is a Doula and hypnobirthing teacher, and lives in Brighton with her husband and their two children. Laura embarked on a huge career change in 2016 to become a hypnobirthing teacher. Experiencing prenatal anxiety herself led her to hypnobirthing as a way to prepare for a positive pregnancy and birth.

Laura teaches her courses in-person and virtually, and is passionate about how important antenatal education is. She is also the Teacher Training Coordinator at The Mindful Birth Group® where she trains and supports their UK network of teachers, providing the first fully inclusive and impartial hypnobirthing course for both vaginal and Caesarean births.

She is passionate about birth rights, the powerful mind-body connection, and continuity of care, and also has a special interest in pregnancy after loss and pregnancy through surrogacy.

www.hellobabybrighton.com

hellobaby_brighton

Tracy Law is a Birth Trauma Counsellor.

As a mother of three and a former midwife with over 35 years of experience, Tracy now specialises in perinatal care, walking alongside families in their healing journeys through pregnancy, birth, and early parenthood. When she is not providing care, you'll find her sea swimming, practicing yoga, or exercising to stay grounded and invigorated. Tracy also loves exploring new countries in her small caravan, discovering hidden gems and creating lifelong memories. Whether in her professional or personal life, she embraces every moment with passion and an open heart.

Tracy is founder of Birth Trauma Resolution Brighton and offers solution focused treatment around any birth trauma experienced by women, men and health professionals and now this is available online she sees women from all over the world!

www.birthtraumaresolutionbrighton.com

@birthtraumaresolution

Dr Jenna Macciochi, is an immunologist specializing in the intersection of nutrition, movement, mind-body practices and lifestyle with the immune system in health and disease. Jenna is a Senior Lecturer in Immunology at The University of Sussex and a fitness instructor and health coach. She is the author of two seminal books *Immunity: The Science of Staying Well* (Harper Collins, 2020) and *Your Blueprint for Strong Immunity* (Yellow Kite, 2022). As a mother of twins and a keen home cook, she brings a personal and realistic touch to her scientifically-baked advice.

www.drjennamacciochi.com

dr_jenna_macciochi

Birth stories

Specialists

Thanks to Dr Georgina Wilson MBChB FRCA for checking through Chapter 5: Different types of anaesthetics for your C-section operation.

References

1. Dr Chrissie Yu (2024). *UK C-Section Rates 2023: Stats, Perspectives & Guidance 2023.* [online] Dr Chrissie Yu. Available at: www.chrissieyu. com/c-section-rates-statistics-uk-global/#:~:text=Sometimes%20this%20 is%20by%20choice

2. NHS Digital (2023). *Maternity Services Monthly Statistics, January 2023, Experimental Statistics.* [online] NDRS. Available at: digital.nhs.uk/dataand-information/publications/statistical maternity-services-monthlystatistics/ january-2023-experimental-statistics

3. Author ID: PE (2021). Vaginal birth following Caesarean Section (VBAC). [online] (8). Available at: www.wwl.nhs.uk/media/.leaflets/617fe9 4083a131.34062713.pdf#:~:text=What%20are%20the%20risks%20 from%20VBAC%3F&text=There%20is%20a%20chance%20you,in%20 100%20women%20(20%25) Leaflet reference: Obs 028.

4. www.npeu.ox.ac.uk (n.d.). *Outcome of Planned Vaginal Birth after Caesarean (VBAC) at Home | NPEU.* [online] Available at: www.npeu.ox.ac.uk/research/ projects/113-birthplace-vbac-at-home

5. March of Dimes | PeriStats (2021). (n.d.). *Total Cesarean Deliveries: United States.* [online] Available at: www.marchofdimes.org/peristats/data?reg=99 &top=8&stop=86&lev=1&slev=1&obj=9&dv=ms

6. Mahoney, K., Heidel, R.E. and Olewinski, L. (2022). Prevalence and normalization of stress urinary incontinence in female strength athletes. *The Journal of Strength & Conditioning Research.* [online] p.10. DOI: pubmed. ncbi.nlm.nih.gov/36930880/

7. Hoeksema, H., De Vos, M., Verbelen, J., Pirayesh, A. and Monstrey, S. (2013). Scar management by means of occlusion and hydration: A comparative study of silicones versus a hydrating gel-cream. *Burns,* 39(7), pp.1437–1448. DOI. Available at: doi.org/10.1016/j.burns.2013.03.025

8. Keag, O.E., Norman, J.E. and Stock, S.J. (2018). Long-term risks and benefits associated with cesarean delivery for mother, baby, and subsequent pregnancies: Systematic review and meta-analysis. *PLOS Medicine.* [online] 15(1), p.e1002494. DOI. Available at: doi.org/10.1371/journal. pmed.1002494

9. Friedman, B. (2012). Conservative treatment for female stress urinary incontinence: simple, reasonable and safe. *Canadian Urological Association journal = Journal de l'Association des urologues du Canada.* [online] 6(1), pp.61–3. DOI: 10.5489/cuaj.12021

10. Perera, J., Kirthinanda, D.S., Wijeratne, S. and Wickramarachchi, T.K. (2014). Descriptive cross sectional study on prevalence, perceptions, predisposing

factors and health seeking behaviour of women with stress urinary incontinence. *BMC Women's Health*, 14(1). DOI. Available at: bmcwomenshealth.
biomedcentral.com/articles/10.1186/1472-6874-14-78

11. Moossdorff-Steinhauser, H.F.A., Berghmans, B.C.M., Spaanderman,
M.E.A. and Bols, E.M.J. (2021). Urinary incontinence 6 weeks to 1 year
post-partum: prevalence, experience of bother, beliefs, and help-seeking
behavior. *International Urogynecology Journal*. DOI. Available at: doi.
org/10.1007/s00192-020-04644-3

12. Holst, K. and Wilson, P.D. (1988). The prevalence of female urinary incontinence and reasons for not seeking treatment. *The New Zealand Medical
Journal*. [online] 101(857), pp.756–758. Available at: pubmed.ncbi.nlm.nih.
gov/3263595/

13. Espino, D.V., Palmer, R.F., Miles, T.P., Mouton, C.P., Lichtenstein, M.J. and
Markides, K.P. (2003). Prevalence and Severity of Urinary Incontinence
in Elderly Mexican-American Women. *Journal of the American Geriatrics
Society*, 51(11), pp.1580–1586. DOI. Available at: pubmed.ncbi.nlm.nih.
gov/14687387/

14. Yildiz P, Ayers S and Phillips L (2017). The prevalence of posttraumatic
stress disorder in pregnancy and after birth: A systematic review and
meta-analysis. *Journal of Affective Disorders 15*, 208, 634–645. DOI:
10.1016/j.jad.2016.10.009

15. Acele, E.Ö. and Karaçam, Z. (2011). Sexual problems in women during the first
postpartum year and related conditions. *Journal of Clinical Nursing*, 21(7–8),
pp.929–937. DOI. Available at: doi.org/10.1111/j.1365-2702.2011.03882.x

16. Pelvic Exercises. (2011). *Prolapse and Sex – What Women Want to Know*.
[online] Available at: https://www.pelvicexercises.com.au/prolapse-sex/

17. Hinterleitner, L., Kiss, H. and Ott, J. (2021). The impact of cesarean section
on female fertility: A narrative review. *Clinical and Experimental Obstetrics
& Gynecology*, 48(4), p.781. DOI. Available at: doi.org/10.31083/j.
ceog4804125

18. Vissers, J., Wouter J. K., Hehenkamp, C.B., Lambalk and Judith A.F. Huirne
(2020). Post-Caesarean section niche-related impaired fertility: hypothetical
mechanisms. *Human Reproduction*, 35(7), pp.1484–1494. DOI. Available at:
doi.org/10.1093/humrep/deaa094

Index